21c

# Perfumes and Cosmetics
in the
Ancient World

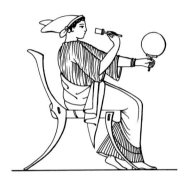

## The Israel Museum
## Jerusalem

Weisbord Exhibition Pavilion
November 1989

Curator-in-charge: Michal Dayagi-Mendels
Catalogue design: Ora Yafeh

Exhibition design: Elisheva Yarhi
English translation: Inna Pommerantz
Illustrations: Florica Vainer
Map: Rivka Myers
Assistant curator: Carine Cohn

Photographs: Nahum Slapak;
David Harris (pp. 11, 87);
Reuben and Edith Hecht Museum,
Haifa University, Haifa (p. 30);
Musée du Louvre (p. 31 above, p. 45
above, p. 92);
The Metropolitan Museum of Art (p. 39);
Landesmuseum Trier (p. 79);
Gabi Laron, Institute of Archeology,
The Hebrew University, Jerusalem (p. 107);
Garo Nalbandian (p. 129);
Zev Radovan (p. 127)

Typesetting: Graph Press Ltd., Jerusalem
Mechanicals: Margalit Bassan
Color separations: Reprocolor Ltd., Tel Aviv
Plates: Tafsar Ltd., Jerusalem
Printed by Sabinsky Press Ltd., Tel Aviv
Bound by Keter Publishing House
Jerusalem Ltd.

Catalogue no. 305
ISBN 965 278 058 8

# Perfumes and Cosmetics
# in the
# Ancient World

Michal Dayagi-Mendels

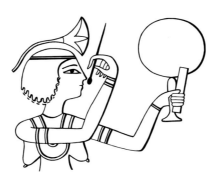

## Catalogue by courtesy of

Dr. A. Giniger
Taya Israel Cosmetic Co. Ltd.
Robert and Janice Atkin

## Exhibition by courtesy of

Canadian friends who love the Israel Museum
Cecile and Leon Fiszman
Dorothy and Albert Gellman
Hermann Mayer
Suzanne and Simon Sigal
Joyce and Edward Strauss
The Promised Land – Movers International Ltd.

## Lenders to the Exhibition

Archaeological Staff Officer of Judaea and Samaria
Bible Lands Museum, Jerusalem (Elie Borowski Collection)
Ella Brummer, New York
Herbert Cahn, Basel
Maurice M. Cohen, Miami
Ecole Biblique, Jerusalem
Eretz Israel Museum, Tel Aviv
Galerie Nefer, Zurich
Father Godfrey, Jerusalem
Israel Department of Antiquities and Museums
Abraham Levy, Jerusalem
Sam Levy, Lisbon
The Masada Archaeological Expedition, Hebrew University,
Jerusalem
Leo Mildenberg, Zurich
Museum of Regional and Mediterranean Archaeology,
Gan Hashlosha
Reuben and Edith Hecht Museum, University of Haifa, Haifa
Jonathan Rosen, New York
Spaer Family, Jerusalem
Louis Warschaw, Los Angeles
Wilfrid Israel Museum Oriental Art and Studies, Kibbutz Hazorea
Anonymous lenders

# Contents

6 Preface
8 Introduction

13 Body Care
35 Facial Care and Makeup
59 Hair and Hair-styles
89 Perfume Production
113 The Spice Trade
125 Spices in Funerary Customs

134 Ownership Credits
135 List of Illustrations
137 Abbreviations
137 Bibliography

This publication accompanies the exhibition "Perfumes and Cosmetics in the Ancient World" at the Israel Museum, Jerusalem. The exhibition is organized in six sections, and presents implements and accessories that were used for facial and hair care, body grooming, perfume production and marketing, as well as numerous perfume bottles which have been found in burials.

In this catalogue, as in the exhibition, we have chosen to focus on the functional aspects of cosmetics known to us from Palestine and the neighboring countries, from the third millennium BCE and until the Roman period. We discuss here mainly the personal uses of cosmetics, touching only slightly on ritual or ceremonial aspects. We have chosen to emphasize chiefly what is known about this subject from Palestine, and to illuminate the findings with the often much more extensive information extant in other countries. For the early periods, we have drawn widely on Egyptian sources, since Egypt is known to have greatly influenced the Canaanite world. For the First Temple period, our knowledge derives mainly from the Bible, although that information concerns mainly ritual aspects of spices and cosmetics. On the other hand, Jewish sources of the Second Temple and Talmudic periods are rich in information on many aspects of personal care, and we have been able to draw directly on these sources.

The objects that have been chosen to illustrate our discussion have not been selected for their beauty, but primarily for the uses that were made of them. We therefore present them not in their chronological or artistic contexts, but in classifications according to their presumed contents or functions. For purposes of demonstration, the text is accompanied by illustrations from wall paintings, pottery vases, and reliefs. Frequently we have had to guess the use of a vessel by its shape and dimensions, as in the case of the stone cosmetic palettes in which traces of paint are seen as evidence that they were used for grinding minerals. Unfortunately, in most of the vessels the original contents have not been preserved, and in those cases where sediments have remained, they were seldom analyzed.

Having excluded the subject of ritual from our discussion, we have also not considered those plants and resins used solely for incense, since incense served mainly for ritual purposes, though it was also used in burial practices and for domestic purposes.

I would like to express my deep gratitude towards all those who gave of their time and knowledge for the sake of this exhibition and catalogue. While it is not possible to mention all their names, certain individuals and organizations are deserving of special recognition: L.Y. Rahmani shared with me his wide knowledge of burial practices in the Second Temple period; Ronny Reich of the Israel Department of Antiquities and Museums reviewed the chapter "Body Care" and made a number of important suggestions regarding the topic of bathing; Uza Zevulun and Gusta Lehrer Jacobson of the Eretz Israel Museum and Meir Ben-Dov of Jerusalem offered important advice in our many conversations;

Joseph Geiger and Hannah Cotton of the Hebrew University brought to my attention information found in papyri from Masada regarding the *aparsemon* (balsam); Zeev Aizenshtat of the Hebrew University kindly conducted chemical tests on the residual sediments of vessels, and provided us with his findings.

Most of the items on display are from the collections of the Israel Department of Antiquities and Museums, though other institutions, museums and private collectors have kindly opened their collections to us. Without their generosity, the exhibition would not have been possible.

Special thanks are also due to the friends of the Israel Museum abroad, who joined in the effort by bringing some of the items for the exhibition with them to Israel: Leo Mildenberg and Jacqueline Weil of Zurich, and Lawrence Cartier of London.

International Flavors and Fragrances (E.A.M.E.), Holland, graciously contributed by developing the essences.

Finally, I would like to thank my co-workers at the Israel Museum: the dedicated team of the Laboratories, for restoring the items and preparing them for the exhibit; the staff of the Exhibition Department, for the attractive design of the display; the staff of the Photography Department, for the skillful photographs of the objects; and the staff of the Publications Department, for its devoted efforts towards the publication of this catalogue. Special thanks are due to Vivianne Barsky, who gave the finishing touches to the English manuscript. I am also indebted to my colleagues, the archaeologists, and above all Yael Israeli, Chief Curator for Archaeology, who supported me throughout all the stages of this project; Ruth Goshen-Oved, who was of particular assistance with the collection and organization of material for the chapter "The Spice Trade"; Claire Kokia; and, last but not least, Edna Peretz, whose tireless efforts enabled us to see the opening of this exhibition. To all these people, my warmest appreciation.

M. D-M.

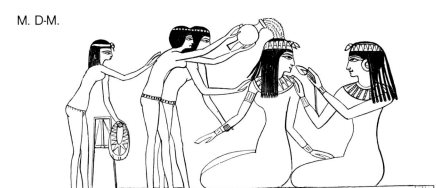

Lady being groomed by her maidservants, Egypt, New Kingdom

Cosmetics have been popular since the dawn of civilization. Their use originated in the ancient East, and then spread westward, first to Greece and afterwards to Rome. Until the advent of Christianity cosmetics were widely used, at times to excess, but the Christian conception, which stressed the life of the spirit and rejected the pleasures of the body, led to a decline in the demand for cosmetics and perfumes, although in the East the Arabs continued to enjoy their use. In medieval Europe, cosmetics and perfumes were associated with the exoticism of the East, and from the Renaissance on they again became popular, mainly among men and women of the European aristocracy.

Since cosmetics are still in wide use today, it is interesting to compare the attitudes, customs and beliefs related to them in ancient times to those of our own day and age. Today, cosmetics are used both to preserve freshness of complexion and body skin, and to make oneself fragrant for the pleasure of others. In antiquity, however, at least at the outset, cosmetics served magico-religious and healing purposes. To propitiate the gods, cosmetics were applied to their statues, and also to the faces of their attendants. From this, in the course of time, developed the custom of personal use, to enhance the beauty of the face, and to conceal defects.

The most extensive information on everything to do with personal hygiene and cosmetics in the third and second millennia BCE comes from Egypt. Written and pictorial descriptions as well as rich archaeological finds, all show how important body care and aesthetic appearance were in the lives of the Egyptian aristocracy. For example, bathing for pleasure was common practice in Egypt, while among other peoples of the ancient East it was limited mainly to religious requirements, although it also had hygienic associations. The use of oils and ointments was prevalent, then as now, to protect the face and body from sun, dust, and the dryness of the Eastern climate. These perfumed oils and ointments were not regarded as luxuries and were used by men and women of all strata of the population. There exists a document which records that Pharaoh Seti I increased the allocation of oils to his army, and it is also known that during the reign of Rameses III the grave diggers of Thebes went on strike in protest against a decline in the quality of the food and the quantity of the oils supplied to them.

The Hebrews used ointments in the Temple and in the coronation ceremonies, as recorded in the description of the anointing of David: "Then Samuel took the horn of oil and anointed him in the midst of his brethren" (1 Samuel, 16:13). The Bible makes no mention of other uses of cosmetics during the First Temple period, but for the Second Temple period we have evidence of the use of cosmetics for secular purposes. In the course of time this custom presumably became so widespread and commonplace that in the Talmud it is said that a husband is obliged to give his wife ten dinars for her cosmetic needs (Babyl. *Ketuboth*, 66b).

The cosmetic preparations included powders, ointments, perfumes and fragrant oils, which were produced from various plants and resins mixed with vegetable oil or animal fat. Because of their high price, all these cosmetic substances were marketed in small quantities. This led to the development of an entire industry manufacturing tiny containers, which became beautifully fashioned luxury articles in their own right. These containers were made of suitable materials such as stone and alabaster, which keep their contents cool. In Egypt, most of the containers were made of stone, while in Greece and Rome they were made of pottery and ornamented with fine paintings. When the technique of glass-blowing developed in the first century BCE, the perfume industry immediately adopted this light-weight and impermeable material for making perfume containers. Most of our information about perfume containers comes from reliefs and wall paintings in Egyptian tombs and from Greek and Roman vase paintings.

Many perfume containers have been found in tombs, having been offered as funerary gifts to the dead or buried with them as cherished personal belongings. The large quantities of perfume bottles found indicate that they were also brought there to freshen the air in the tombs during burial. The function of perfumes and spices in burial will be discussed in the chapter "Spices in Funerary Customs."

Great importance was attached to the care of the hair in ancient times. Long hair has always been considered a mark of beauty, and kings, nobles and dignitaries grew their hair long and kept it well-groomed and cared for. Ordinary people and slaves usually wore their hair short, mainly for hygienic reasons, since they could not afford to invest in the kind of care that long hair required. The art of hairstyling and hair care reached its apogee during the Roman period, as can be learned from the numerous heads of statues which have survived from that time.

The composition and manufacture of cosmetics has always been an important and intriguing subject. Latent in perfumes are powers of seduction and illusion and they are capable of arousing either tender feelings or aggressiveness. Perfumes can be used both to attract and to repel. The various fragrances combined in perfumes – some fresh and light, others sweet and heavy, yet others exotic and aphrodisiac – may be mixed in an almost endless variety of combinations, an art which requires both imagination and refinement of taste. People working in this field had to be endowed, then as now, not only with skill and knowledge, but also with a memory for fragrances, and an ability to identify them and distinguish their combinations. The perfumers of antiquity guarded the secrets of their trade closely, passing on their skills from father to son. Perfumes and spices were very expensive and were kept together with silver and gold. For example, we read in the Bible that when King Hezekiah of Judah received royal guests from Babylon, "he showed them all his treasure house, the silver, and the gold, and the spices, the precious ointment, the house of his armor and all that was found in his treasures" (2 Kings, 20:13). Today, when many of the modern scents are produced by chemists in laboratories, their prices have fallen considerably. In ancient times, however, all perfumes were made from

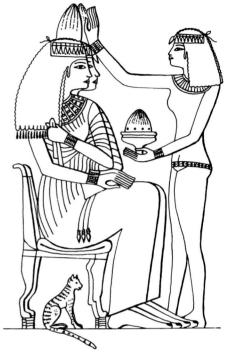

Maidservant applying fragrant ointment to her mistress's hair, Egypt

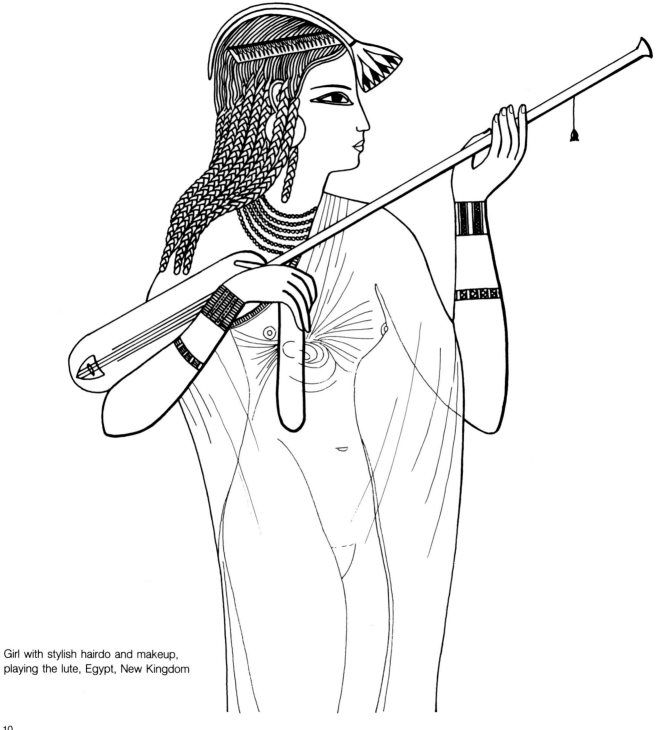

Girl with stylish hairdo and makeup,
playing the lute, Egypt, New Kingdom

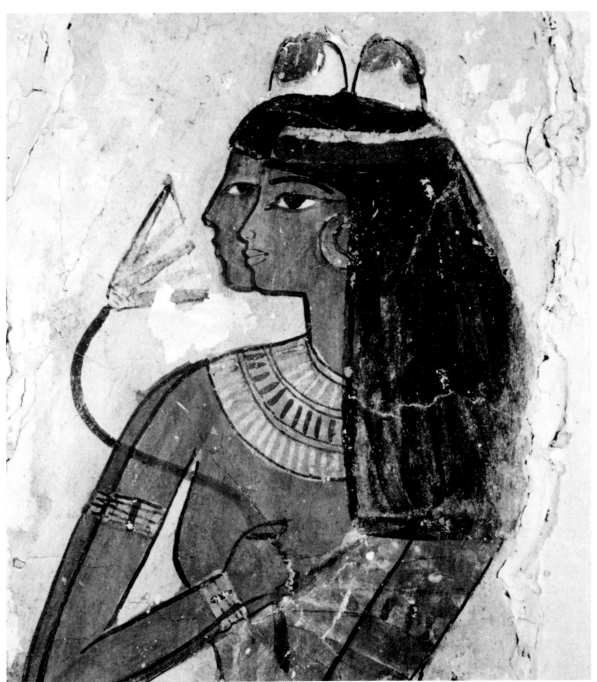

Fashionable ladies attending a banquet, wall painting, Egypt, New Kingdom

11

natural materials, some of which were rare and brought from afar, and some of a kind that could be produced only in tiny quantities, and hence their costliness. Further on we will discuss ancient methods of producing perfumes, and the perfume workshop that has been excavated at En Gedi. A special discussion will be devoted to the famous balsam (Hebrew *aparsemon*) which was grown in this area and was one of the most sought after perfumes in the ancient world. Ancient sources provide some information about the components of perfumes, as well as recipes for making them. The classical authors Theophrastus, Pliny and Dioscorides have left especially detailed descriptions of the cultivation of perfume plants and of the production of perfumes and ointments from them. Other classical sources emphasize the widespread use of perfumes in 6th-century BCE Greece, and their central place in cultural and social life. Perfume shops functioned as meeting-places for all strata of the population. Philosophers, statesmen, artists and writers who wished to discuss matters of state would gather in such places, and their presence attracted many others. Some citizens, however, frowned on such self-indulgence. The renowned statesman and poet, Solon, for example, prohibited the sale of perfumes and ointments in his state, and the rulers of Sparta banished the perfumers from their city. The most lavish consumers of perfumes were the Romans, who perfumed each part of their body with a different scent, sprinkled perfume on their guests at banquets, and even perfumed the walls of their bathrooms. In the houses of the wealthy the beds on which they slept or the couches on which they reclined during meals were filled with fragrant dried flowers. Pliny criticized this excessive use of scent and the waste of money, commenting that despite their costliness – sometimes more than 400 denarii an ounce – perfumes gave pleasure only to others, since the user himself could not smell them at all (Pliny, *Nat. Hist.*, XIII: 20–22).

Using scent was common practice in Eretz Israel too during the Second Temple period, and not only among women. The Talmud mentions the priests of the Abtinas family, who had the monopoly on preparing incense for the Temple. They refused to let others share in the knowledge of their craft, fearing it might be used for profane purposes. Also, to prevent suspicion that they themselves might be exploiting their skills profanely, their wives were forbidden to use scent, even when they were brides (Babyl. *Yoma*, 38a). It is also recorded that they took strict precautions to protect the secrets of their craft and to prevent forgeries. Perfumes were sold in shops located in the market, which was often a meeting-place for harlots. By the nature of things, the harlots needed especially large quantities of perfumes (*Shemoth Rabbah*, 43:7). To this day, there is a narrow street in the Old City of Jerusalem that is called "The Spice Market."

The plants and resins used for producing the perfumes had to be brought from distant places, mainly from South Arabia and the Far East. To facilitate their transport, extensive trading networks developed, and the countries that the caravan routes traversed enjoyed great economic prosperity as a result. We shall discuss mainly the trade routes to Palestine, and the best-known and most popular plants transported along these routes.

# Body Care

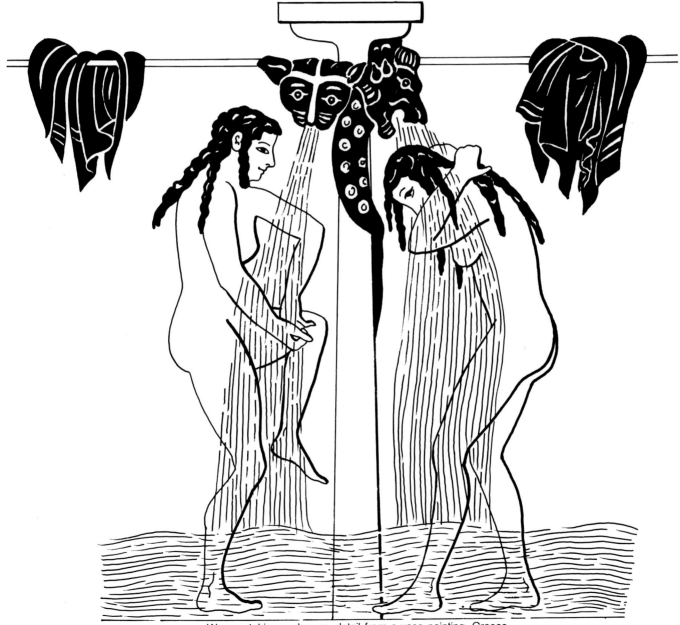

Women taking a shower, detail from a vase painting, Greece

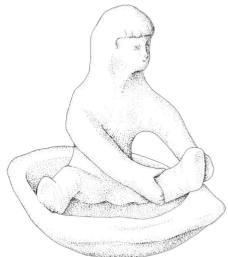

Figurine of a woman bathing in a tub, pottery, Akhziv, 7th century BCE

In the hot, dry climate of the East, washing the body and anointing it with oil were hygienic necessities of the first order. Obviously, the frequency of bathing was influenced not only by the availability of water, but also by social status. Wealthy people could of course pay stricter attention to their body hygiene than could members of the poorer classes. Generally speaking, people of the ancient East contented themselves with washing only the face, hands, and feet, although in Egypt daily bathing appears to have been the rule. The Babylonians, on the other hand, washed the entire body mainly in preparation for religious festivals. In the Bible, too, bathing is mentioned mostly in connection with ritual purity. It was also the rule among the Hebrews to bathe after a sickness or a war, and women were instructed to purify themselves from menstrual uncleanness.

Washing the hands was one of the practices common to all peoples of the ancient East. It was customary to wash the hands on rising in the morning and before meals, and mostly also after meals. In the New Testament we read that "The Pharisees, and all the Jews, do not eat unless they wash their hands" (Mark, 7:3) and in the Talmud it is said that one must wash one's hands every morning and evening and before prayer (Babyl. *Shabbath*, 109a).

In ancient Greece, banquet guests washed their hands in perfumed warm water and wiped them on a common towel. In the East, no special vessels for rinsing the hands are known, with the exception of Egypt, where spouted vessels have been found next to basins. These vessels are frequently depicted on reliefs and in paintings, where they are seen standing under the table. They are known from the 3rd and 2nd millennia BCE and were mostly made of bronze and at times of alabaster and pottery.

Another prevalent custom in the ancient East was washing the feet. This custom is mentioned in the Bible as part of the conventions of hospitality, obliging the host to offer his guests water to wash the dust of the journey off their feet. Abraham observed this custom when the three angels came to visit him: "Let a little water be fetched and wash your feet" (Genesis, 18:4) and so did Lot (Genesis, 19:2). David, too, commanded Uriah: "Go down to your house and wash your feet" (2 Samuel, 11:8). It is probably in the context of this custom that the footbaths known from Eretz Israel in the Iron Age should be interpreted. These are pottery basins, mostly oval, with a footrest in them and a spout at the bottom for emptying the dirty water. Footbaths like these have been found at Samaria, Megiddo, Tell en-Nasbeh, Lachish and elsewhere from the 8th–7th centuries BCE. Similar basins were in use among Palestinian Arabs for washing the feet before prayer. In the bathrooms of 1st-century houses in the upper city of Jerusalem, stone installations have been found which probably served as footbaths of the kind mentioned in the Mishnah (*Yadaim*, 4:1).

According to Jewish literary sources it was one of the wife's duties to wash the feet, hands, and face of her husband, even if there were servants in the house (Babyl.

*Ketuboth*, 61a). This washing was intended to be enjoyable and was done with hot water, in contrast to the hasty washing in the mornings, for which cold water was used. After the washing of the feet it was customary to anoint them with oil, as recorded in the New Testament ". . . she has anointed my feet with ointment" (Luke, 7:46).

The ancient Egyptians, as we have mentioned, paid great attention to the cleanliness of the entire body and bathed daily, usually in the morning after rising, and often after meals as well. They attached special importance to washing the statues of the gods, a daily task assigned to the priests. The priests themselves were required to be especially strict about their body cleanliness and had to bathe three times a day. Depictions on sarcophagi and paintings indicate that bathrooms existed in Egypt already in the earliest periods. However, these crumbled together with the dwellings they served, as they were built of perishable mudbrick, unlike the tombs and splendid temples built of lasting stone.

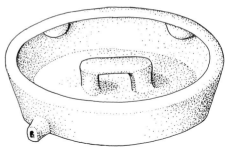

Footbath, pottery, Samaria, 9th–8th centuries BCE

In the tomb of Ruaben, an official of the IInd Dynasty, there is a depiction of a house containing a bathroom. In houses of the XIIth Dynasty excavated at Kahun, bathrooms were uncovered next to the bedrooms, while in houses of the XVIIIth Dynasty at Tell el-Amarna the bathrooms were located at the rear of the house. The bathing was actually more like a shower performed in the bathroom, which contained a large stone slab raised slightly above the floor, with a drain next to it. The bather stood on this stone slab and his servant poured water over him through a sieve. Obviously, such bathrooms existed mainly in palaces and in the homes of the wealthy, and people of lesser means must have washed in a basin or bathed in the river.

In contrast to the Egyptians, the people of Mesopotamia washed the entire body only on festal occasions. The priests washed in running water, in a river or stream, in honor of the divine festivals. The ordinary worshiper also had to wash his body if he wished to approach the god to offer a sacrifice. On special occasions, as after an illness or a war, it was customary among the Babylonians and Assyrians to purify the body by bathing. The common people bathed in the rivers or in the reservoirs in the courtyards, while the notables and wealthy citizens had special bathing installations in their palaces and mansions.

Bathtubs existed also at Mari, where two basins standing on a raised platform were uncovered in one of the rooms of the palace. It has been suggested that one of the two basins was intended for hot water and the other for cold water, or that one basin was for the king and the other for the queen. Paved bathrooms equipped with drains, as well as the remains of a bronze bathtub have been unearthed at Sinjirli in North Syria. Many bathrooms containing bathtubs have also been found in palaces at Crete and Mycenae of the 2nd millennium BCE. In the Neo-Babylonian period (7th–6th centuries BCE), bathrooms in private houses became quite common. Excavations have revealed drainage systems and plastered floors of baked bricks sloping towards the center of the room.

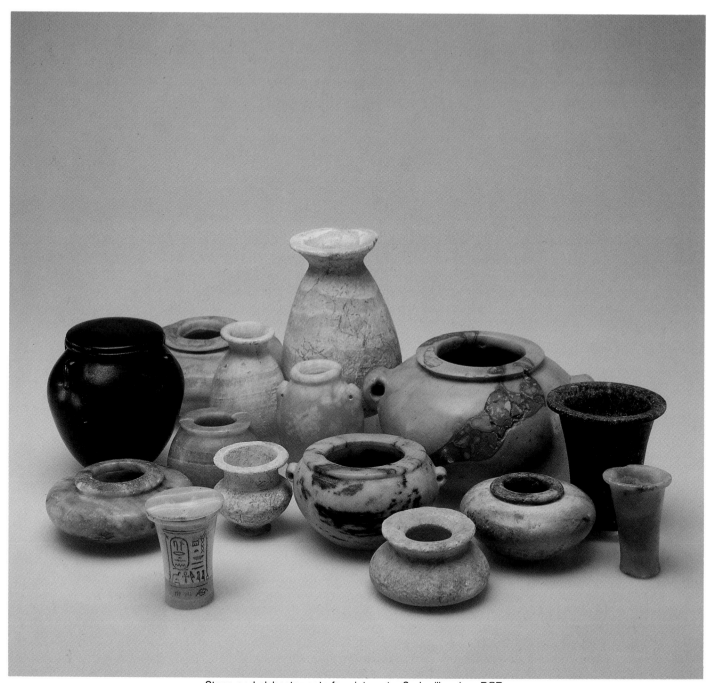

Stone and alabaster pots for ointments, 2nd millennium BCE

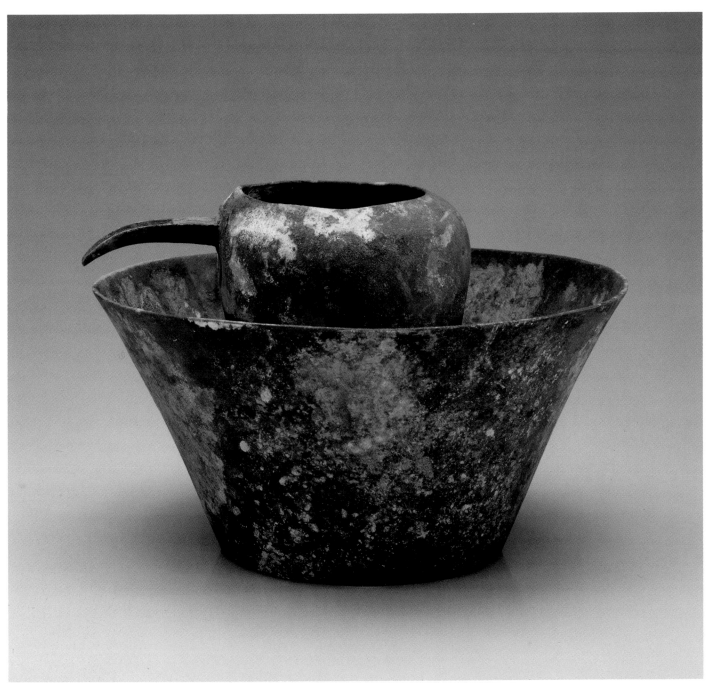

Basin and ewer for washing the hands, bronze, Egypt, Old Kingdom

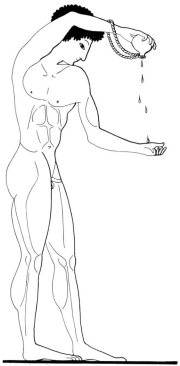

Athlete dribbling oil from an aryballos, detail from a painting on a kylix, Greece, c. 500 BCE

Similar bathrooms existed also in the Assyrian palaces. It appears that the actual washing was done by means of a "shower."

Although bathrooms were a rarity in Palestine until the Hellenistic period, several early examples have been discovered. In the two Egyptian governors' palaces of the second quarter of the 2nd millennium BCE, excavated at Tell el-Ajjul, rooms were found with plastered sloping floors and a drainage system, which are believed to have been bathrooms. In one room in the earlier of these two palaces, excavators found a raised platform with a large jug beside it. The jug was probably used for pouring water over the bather. At Tell Jemmeh, a room excavated in a palace from the Late Canaanite period (13th century BCE) had a drainage system in the floor, and both the floor and the walls were plastered. Another washing installation, consisting of a cistern fitted with an overflow channel, was uncovered at Megiddo in the Late Canaanite stratum. In these bathrooms, washing seems to have been carried out while the bather was standing. However, some washed in a basin or tub, as demonstrated by the 7th-century BCE figurine of a woman washing herself, found in a Phoenician tomb at Akhziv. Another figurine, of a man sitting in a basin while a woman washes him, is known from Cyprus, and belongs to the same period. These shallow basins held a relatively small quantity of water and it would seem that the bather sat in the basin while an attendant poured water over him. Biblical stories imply that it was also customary to wash in enclosed courtyards; thus David could spy Bathsheba washing herself, probably in the courtyard of her house, from the roof of his house (2 Samuel, 11:2). Presumably many people also bathed in streams and springs.

Various vegetal or mineral substances were added to the bathwater in antiquity. Jeremiah (2:22) speaks of washing with niter and vegetable alkali (borit), both of them materials that contain potassium – borit consists of ashes of plants containing potassium, and niter is mineral potassium. The Egyptians added niter and oils mixed with lime to the water, and in Mesopotamia the additive was oil boiled with alkali and clay. While the potassium did indeed dissolve the dirt, it also caused an unpleasant irritation of the skin. According to Pliny, it was the Gauls who invented soap – a mixture of goat fat and vegetal ashes (Pliny, Nat. Hist., XXVIII:191) – but the solid soap that we know today is a European invention of the Middle Ages.

To prevent the skin from drying and cracking after the use of the harsh minerals, and to protect it in the hot, dry climate, it was customary to anoint the body with oil after bathing. Thus we read about Naomi advising her daughter-in-law Ruth: "Wash yourself and anoint yourself and put on your raiment" (Ruth, 3:3). Oiling the body was not considered a luxury and in most countries of the ancient East body oils were regarded as a basic everyday commodity and were used by the majority of the population. Therefore, it was a sign of mourning to refrain from anointing: "be a mourner and put on mourning apparel and do not anoint yourself with oil" (2 Samuel, 14:2).

The Egyptians knew more than 30 different oils and ointments for anointing the skin, and in Persia, too, the various oils and cosmetics were well differentiated, as we read in the story of Esther: "Now when every maiden's turn came to go into the king . . . for so was the period of their beautification accomplished, six months with oil of myrrh and six months with perfumes and ointments for women" (Esther, 2:12)

In the Greek world, the attitude to body cosmetics was very different, mainly because there the need to take care of the body was to a great extent connected with sports, of which ablutions and oiling formed part. Already in the 4th century BCE, the palaestras and gymnasiums where athletes exercised were equipped with bathing facilities, and these were continually improved over the centuries. Before the competition, the athletes would oil their skin and sprinkle it with a powder appropriate for the kind of sport they were doing. This oily layer was removed after the game with a strigil, a scraper made specifically for this purpose. The strigil, the aryballos (oil bottle) and the sponge were part of an athlete's personal equipment. In Greek vase paintings the aryballos is shown hanging from the athlete's wrist while he drips oil from it onto his palm or rubs it onto his body. The strigil, an instrument originally used by athletes, eventually turned into a personal accessory for daily use of men and women. It was customary to hang the strigil on a ring in the bath.

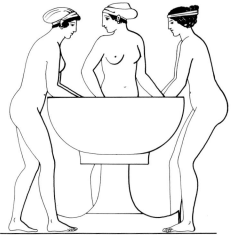

Women washing in a basin,
after a vase painting,
Greece, 5th century BCE

Surprisingly few remains of bathtubs have been found in private houses. Most of our information comes from literary sources and from depictions on vase paintings. Thus Homer, for example, describes preparations for a banquet in a noble house: "And when the maids had bathed them and anointed them with oil . . . . Then a handmaid brought water for the hands in a fair pitcher of gold and poured it over a silver basin for them to wash" (*Odyssey*, IV:49–53). The paintings show bathers in a fountain or women washing themselves in a basin. Footbaths were also used, and in banqueting scenes, they are shown standing under the couches. In Greece, too, anointing the body with oil was a routine matter, often replacing washing or bathing.

In the Hellenistic world, the bathroom became a regular fixture in the homes of the middle classes, as has been shown by various excavations, for instance at Olynthus in Greece. At the same time, baths open to the public at large were established, serving especially those exercising in the palaestras and gymnasiums. Such baths have been discovered at Olympia and Athens as well as other sites. According to Roman authors, the transition from ordinary bathing to the use of elaborate baths, either private or public, occurred in the 2nd century BCE. In these baths the bather sat in a bathtub while an attendant poured hot water over him. The water had been heated in an installation in the adjoining room.

The Romans took over the bathing installations from the Greeks and perfected them further. The Roman baths contained three main units: the *tepidarium* (warm room), the

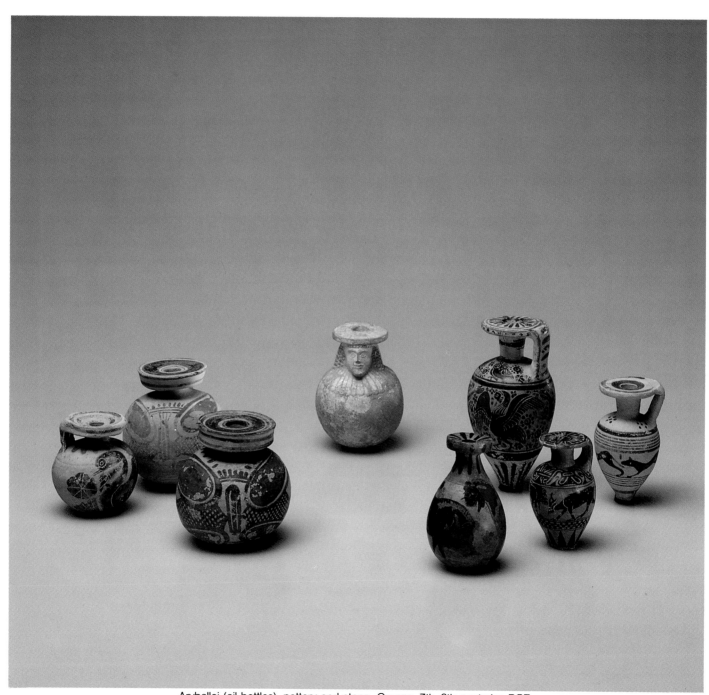

Aryballoi (oil bottles), pottery and stone, Greece, 7th–6th centuries BCE

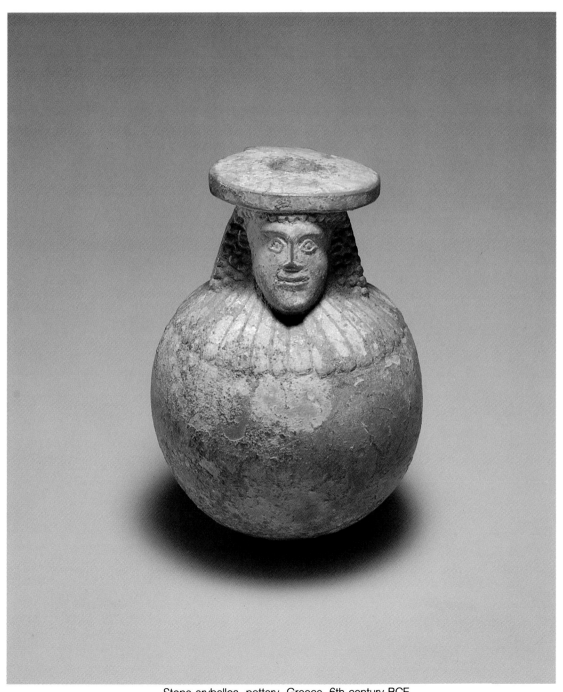

Stone aryballos, pottery, Greece, 6th century BCE

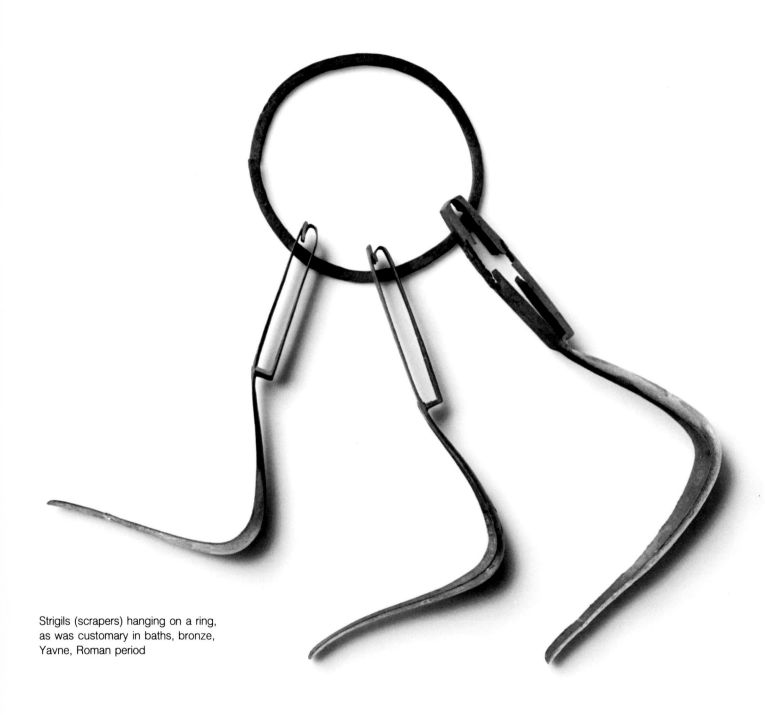

Strigils (scrapers) hanging on a ring,
as was customary in baths, bronze,
Yavne, Roman period

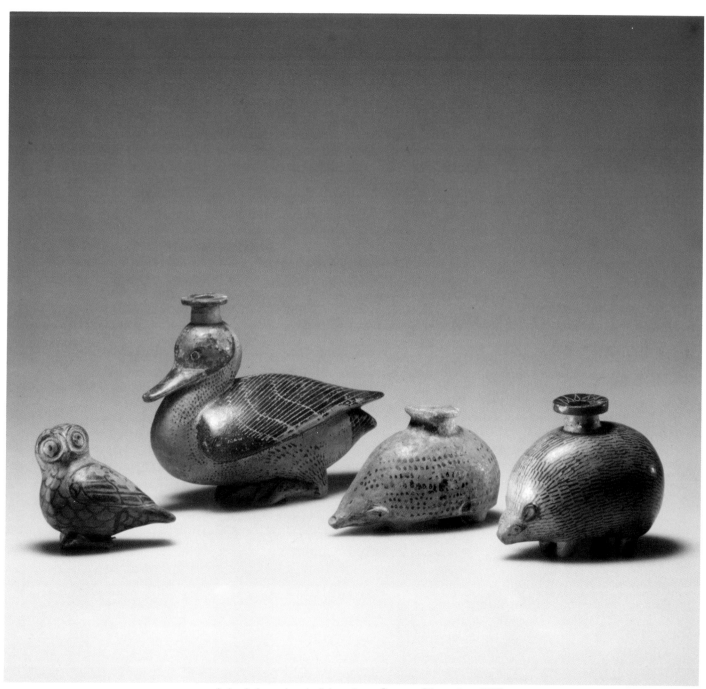

Animal-shaped aryballoi, pottery, Greece, 6th century BCE

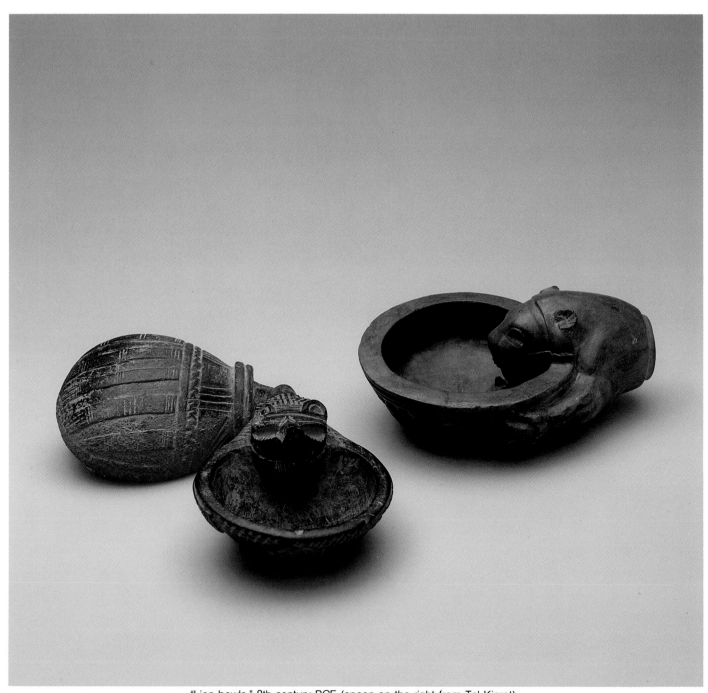

"Lion bowls," 8th century BCE (spoon on the right from Tel Kinrot)

*caldarium* (hot room), and the *frigidarium* (cold room). In the more spacious baths there was usually also a cloakroom and at times a sweating-room, and the most elaborate baths contained a room for anointing the body with oil and another room for wiping it off. The main technical improvement introduced by the Romans was the construction of the hot room floor on low ceramic pillars, making it possible to heat the entire room, including the water in the bathtubs, by the influx of very hot air into the space beneath the floor.

In Rome, going to the baths was a social occasion and a central part of everyday life. The Romans regarded bathing not only as a hygienic necessity, but also as a form of entertainment, which went on for many hours. They erected many public baths which were open to all. Some of these were very large, and could serve up to two thousand people, like the Baths of Caracalla and Diocletian in Rome. On entering, the patron took off his clothes and deposited them for safekeeping. He then proceeded to the unguent shop where the shelves were stocked with jars of various sizes containing many kinds of unguents and creams, a different unguent for each part of the body. Having made his choice, he moved on to the exercise areas and to the various bathing and steam rooms. After bathing his body was massaged with ointments, either by his personal servant or by a person employed for this task by the baths.

The pampered Roman lady entrusted herself, immediately after her bath, to the hands of her personal staff of maids, headed by the *ornatrix*: one maid was charged with massaging her after the bath; another with rubbing her skin with unguents; a third with the care of her hands and feet; and yet another with plucking out unwanted hairs. When the lady set out for the bath, she took her creams and unguents with her; these were kept in a special box which was prudently placed in a locked cupboard. It is related that Emperor Nero's wife, Poppaea, who was renowned for her extravagance and ostentation, bathed daily in a tub filled with asses' milk to which perfumes had been added.

In some of the public baths uncovered in excavations, double sets of installations have come to light – one for men and one for women. In fact, mixed bathing was the rule until early in the 2nd century CE, when Emperor Hadrian (117–138 CE) issued an edict decreeing separation of the sexes. Henceforth, different hours were allotted in the baths for men and for women. It was customary to visit the public baths in the morning hours, before the main meal of the day.

Under the influence of Hellenistic culture baths began appearing in Palestine too – and not only in the houses of the nobility. At Beth Zur, many plastered bathtubs were uncovered which had an opening near the bottom for draining the water and sometimes a ledge for sitting. At Gezer, too, a structure was excavated which contained plastered stone bathtubs with a drainage opening at the bottom. In Jerusalem, at Qumran, and at other sites, bathing and immersion pools have been found that are presumably connected with

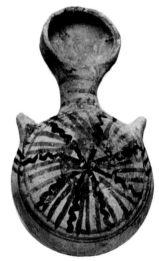

Pilgrim flask for scented oil, pottery, Megiddo, 11th century BCE

Jewish purification laws. In the "Upper City" of Jerusalem, houses of the wealthy from the 1st century CE have been uncovered with remains of bathrooms and bathtubs as well as ritual baths. In Samaria, houses of the Roman period have been excavated, which contained bathrooms with hip-baths or stepped pools.

The earliest Roman baths that have been uncovered in this country are those at Tel Anafa in Galilee and in Herod's palaces at Masada, Herodion, Jericho and Kypros. These were functional buildings, satisfactory for requirements of personal hygiene, but far from the size and magnificence of the famous Roman baths.

Despite the hostility that our ancestors harbored against the Romans, they were capable of appreciating the improvements the latter had introduced into the country, among these the baths: "How fine are the works of this people! They have made streets, they have built bridges, they have erected baths" (Babyl. *Shabbath*, 33b). With the growth of the non-Jewish population in the country, the number of public baths increased, and the custom of visiting them began to be adopted also by the Jews. It is related of Hillel the Elder, who sought to teach his pupils the importance of bathing, that "when he concluded his studies with his disciples . . . they asked him: 'Master, whither are you bound?' He answered them: 'To perform a religious duty . . . to wash in a bath-house'" (*Wayyikra Rabba*, 34:3). However, pious Jews had qualms about visits to the baths, as these were usually decorated with pagan symbols and statues and some baths were even dedicated to some pagan deity. Of Rabban Gamaliel, it is told, that when he was asked why he bathed in the bath of Aphrodite in Akko he answered: "I came not within her limits, she came within mine! They do not say 'Let us make a bath for Aphrodite,' but 'Let us make an Aphrodite as an adornment for the bath'" (Mishnah *Abodah Zarah,* 3:4). In saying this he was in fact expressing the rabbinical permission for Jews to visit public baths, which they had previously refrained from doing for religious reasons.

Literary sources mention public baths which were privately owned (Mishnah *Baba Bathra*, 1:6; 10:7) as well as public baths established by municipal authorities or private philanthropists (Mishnah *Nedarim*, 5:5). Another source lists ten conditions that a town must meet before a scholar was allowed to reside there, one of these being the existence of a public bath (Babyl. *Sanhedrin*, 17b).

The public baths contained a large pool in which all the bathers immersed themselves. Private single bathtubs were also available, for a larger fee. A splendid alabaster bathtub weighing a ton and a half was uncovered in a niche in the *caldarium* (hot room) of the baths in Herod's palace at Kypros near Jericho.

The unguents used for anointing the skin after bathing were composed on a base of vegetable oils, such as olive oil, almond oil, sesame oil and others, or on a base of animal fat, such as fat of geese, sheep, goats, or cattle. To these, various fixative materials were

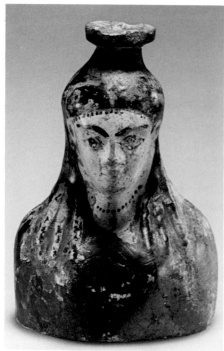

Aryballos in the shape of a woman, pottery, Greece, 6th century BCE

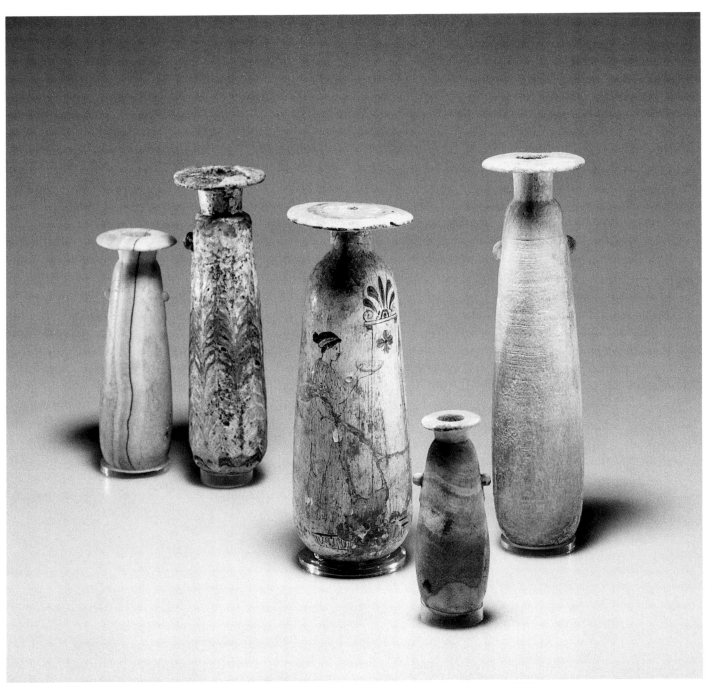

Alabastron bottles, alabaster, pottery and glass, mid-1st millennium BCE

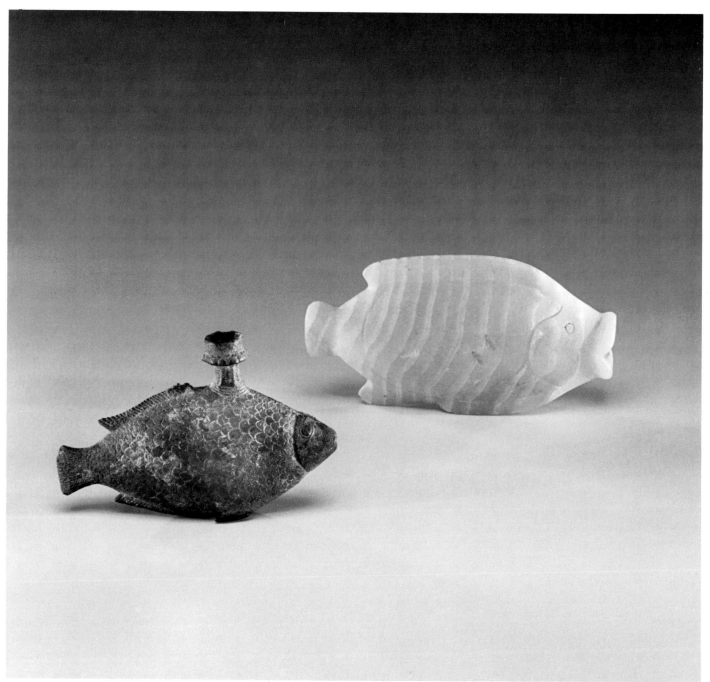

Fish-shaped containers. On the right: alabaster, from Tell el-Ajjul, mid-2nd millennium BCE; on the left: bronze, Greece, c. 600 BCE

added, including milk, honey, and different salts. It is clear that the wealthy treated their skin with precious and perfumed unguents while those with lesser means used oils of inferior quality, such as castor oil. Fragrant resins or aromatic flowers were added to the unguents and oils to give them a sweet scent. Every part of the body was anointed with oil. It is related that the Egyptian queen, Hatshepsut, who reigned in the 15th century BCE, rubbed myrrh on her feet so as to exude a pleasant fragrance; while Seneca, of the 1st century CE, records that Romans of his day used to perfume even the soles of their feet.

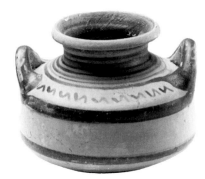

Pyxis (box), pottery, Tel Dan, 14th century BCE

Many recipes for preparing ointments have reached us from ancient Egypt. These have survived on papyri and in inscriptions on temple walls. Fragrant ointments played an important part in rituals, for instance in the ritual of restoring life to divine statues, and in the temples there were special rooms for the preparation of unguents and creams. During the New Kingdom, the priests had an important share in this industry. In Mari too, much information on this subject has been preserved in the extensive collection of documents uncovered in the royal palace. Among these are lists of anointing oils of various kinds and quantities, including fragrant oils that served the needs of the palace. The Bible also mentions the preparation of ointments as part of the activities of the royal court: "This will be the manner of the king . . . he will take your daughters to be perfumers" (1 Samuel, 8:11, 13).

The ointment and oil industry brought in its wake the manufacture of beautiful containers. Boxes and pots of alabaster, faience, ivory, bone, bronze, and pottery have been found in great quantities throughout the ancient East and the Mediterranean region. It is assumed that a large proportion of the small impermeable vessels was used for ointments. It is also believed that receptacles of distinctive shapes were used for this particular purpose.

In Egypt, stone vessels – of granite, diorite, and especially alabaster – were popular already during the Predynastic period. The Egyptian alabaster pots were exported to neighboring countries, including Palestine. The commonest ointment containers were small bowls, spherical or bag-shaped vessels, goblets with everted sides, and amphoriskoi (small jars). Larger alabaster receptacles contained oils for cleansing the body. Ointment containers usually had a narrow neck in relation to the body, so that it could be easily stoppered. Containers with wider necks were closed with a flat stone lid wrapped in leather or fabric, and bound with string for further safety. In addition, there were open alabaster vessels, such as the bowl-shaped, high-footed tazza. This vessel may have been used for mixing the powdered substances with oil or water, or perhaps for offering perfumed oil to participants in banquets. Among the most attractive containers are those in the shape of animals, such as fish, ducks, or hedgehogs, or of human figures. Such vessels were popular in Egypt during the New Kingdom, and also reached Palestine. Of special interest are the alabaster fish from Tell el-Ajjul dating from the first

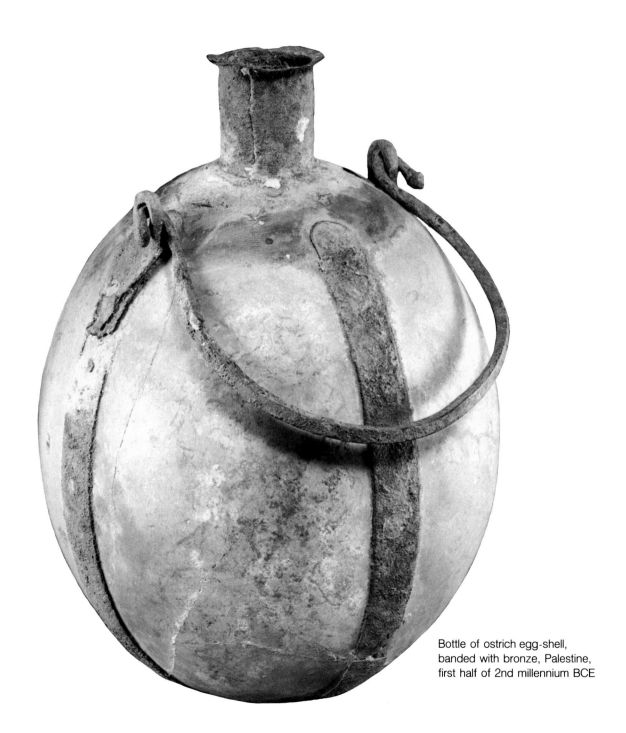

Bottle of ostrich egg-shell,
banded with bronze, Palestine,
first half of 2nd millennium BCE

half of the 2nd millennium BCE and the bronze fish from the middle of the first millennium BCE.

In Egypt, ointment pots were kept in special wooden boxes divided into compartments, or in baskets. These boxes, like the pots themselves, were favored funerary gifts in the tombs of the wealthy, but the containers were stolen or emptied of their precious contents already in antiquity.

In Palestine, pyxides (boxes) of pottery, alabaster, faience, and bone were produced in large quantities during the second half of the 2nd millennium BCE. The local alabaster pyxis is squat, with two handles that are sometimes perforated, and a perforated lid. It was undoubtedly inspired by the Mycenaean pottery pyxis, which was very common in this country during the Late Canaanite period.

Of special interest are the horn-shaped ivory vessels, such as those found in Megiddo, in the treasury of the Late Canaanite palace (13th century BCE). The vessel illustrated here is made of ivory, has a flat base, and is adorned with three gold bands and a female head sprouting a spoon at the end of its neck. Vessels in the shape of ox-horns have been found in Egyptian tombs, often beside other cosmetic vessels. It has been sug-

Cosmetic vessel in the shape of
a human figure, limestone and alabaster, ▷
Egypt, New Kingdom

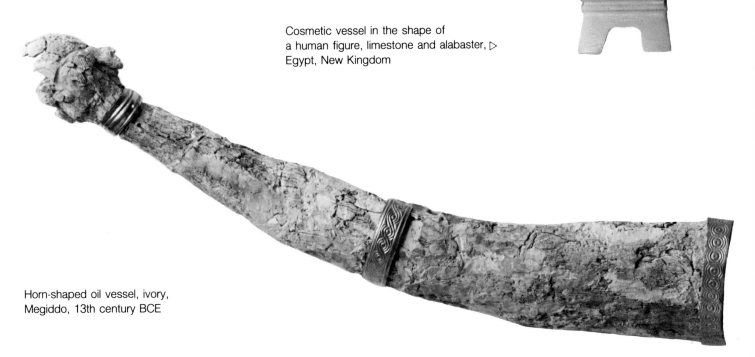

Horn-shaped oil vessel, ivory,
Megiddo, 13th century BCE

31

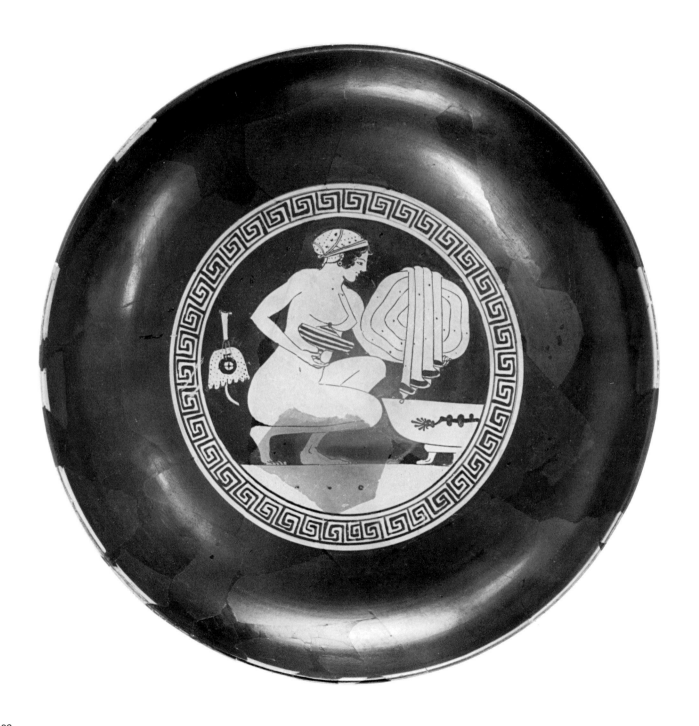

32

gested that these were containers for oil intended for anointing the bodies of pregnant women, while another opinion holds that they had some gynecological function. It is possible that the local horn-shaped pottery vessels from the early Iron Age may have developed from these receptacles. Others wish to identify the horn-shaped vessel with the "horn of oil" used in the anointing of kings: "And Zadok the priest took the horn of oil from the tent and anointed Solomon" (1 Kings, 1:39).

Also belonging to this category are the "lion bowls," which were common in many places in the ancient East: North Syria, Palestine, Anatolia, and Assyria. These bowls, dating

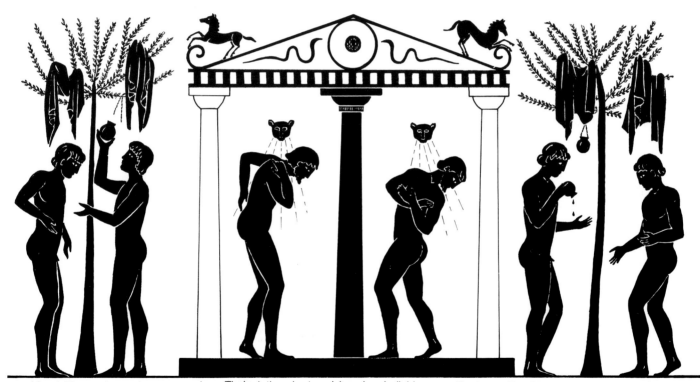

Men taking a shower in a gymnasium. Their clothes (or towels) and aryballoi hang on the trees. Detail from a vase painting, Greece

◁ Woman washing herself. In her left hand she holds a towel, in her right, a plemoche; behind her hang a strigil, an aryballos, and a sponge. Painting on a kylix, attributed to the painter Triptolemos, Greece, 470 BCE

from the 9th–7th centuries BCE, are mostly made of steatite and rarely of ivory, faience, or pottery. Their characteristic feature is the lion's head rising above the rim of the bowl, which is clasped between the lion's forepaws. A horizontal tube emerges from the bowl and is often combined with the lion's head. The bottom of the bowl is decorated with a human hand, a cross design, or a leaf design. The tube was probably fitted to a skin or pottery receptacle from which the liquid could be poured into the bowl, similarly to the lentil-shaped pilgrim flasks from the early Iron Age, which had a rim widening into a bowl. It has been suggested that the "lion bowls" were used in cult ceremonies for libations or drinking. According to another opinion they were used for incense burning, even though no traces of soot have been found on them. However, it is possible that these bowls were used for perfumed oil contained in the receptacle that was attached to the bowl. Presumably, this precious liquid was used for anointing the body, and whatever remained of it in the bowl after use could be returned to the receptacle by tilting the bowl.

Ostrich eggs, which were used as containers for liquids in the 3rd and 2nd millennia BCE, seem to have also served to hold perfumed oils, because of the impermeability of the shell and the fact that, in contrast to pottery, it does not absorb odors. The finest example of these is probably the ostrich egg illustrated here, to which a bronze neck and handle have been added by means of a bronze band.

A wide range of beautiful pottery vessels for cosmetics is known from the classical world. Here, potters and painters were given the opportunity of combining functionality with captivating beauty. The smooth finish of the vessels ensured their impermeability and reduced the absorption of odors by the clay. The aryballos (oil bottle) the alabastron and the pyxis (box), as well as other vessels, were exported by the merchants of Athens and Corinth throughout the Mediterranean region.

The aryballos was the typical oil container that began to appear in Greece in the 7th century BCE. A passage from Homer indicates its importance already at this time: "Her mother gave her also soft olive oil in a flask of gold, that she and her maidens might have it for the bath" (*Odyssey*, VI:79–80). The aryballos, which was originally shaped like an amphoriskos, came in the course of time to be made in a wide variety of forms, including a woman's bust and various animal shapes. Another vessel for cosmetics was the lekanis, a shallow bowl with a lid and two horizontal handles. This vesssel, which began to be produced in Greece in the 6th century BCE became highly popular in the 5th–4th centuries BCE, for instance as a wedding-gift for women. Another cosmetic container was the plemoche, a bowl on a high foot, with a rim folded inwards and a lid. This vessel appears frequently in vase paintings of the 5th century BCE in scenes of bathing women, often next to an alabastron, which was also used for oils and perfumes. The relatively large size of this vessel indicates that it contained a low-grade product, perhaps a diluted perfume for use after bathing.

# Facial Care and Makeup

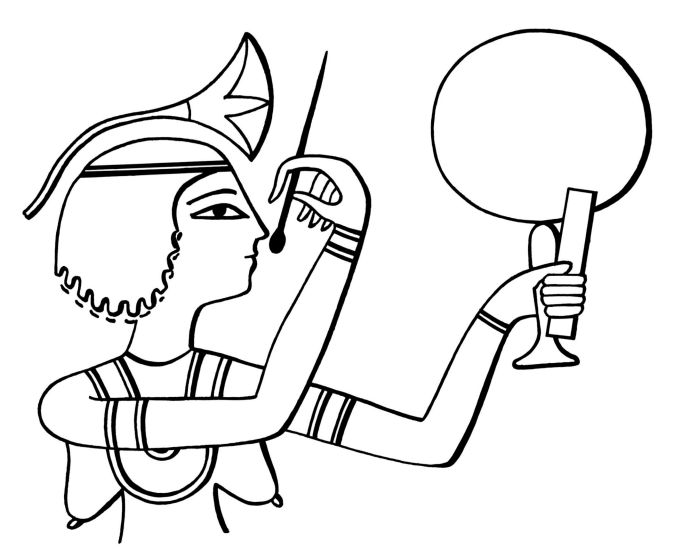

Woman coloring her lips in front of a mirror,
painting on papyrus, Egypt, New Kingdom

The desire to improve and embellish facial appearance has existed since the dawn of civilization, and the practice of making up the face may be traced back to the earliest periods. It has its origins in magic and ritual, and we know that it was customary to cover the statues of gods with unguents and to make up their faces in order to lend them a semblance of life. In the course of time, however, this custom extended to the life of the individual, for aesthetic and medical purposes, and was commonly practiced by both men and women.

Very early evidence of the use of facial makeup has reached us from ancient Egypt. This includes cosmetic utensils and materials as well as numerous written records and artistic depictions of the subject. Paintings on tomb-walls and on papyri, as well as reliefs on sarcophagi and in tombs, give us concrete illustrations of the ways Egyptian women took care of their faces and applied their makeup. The eyes, then as now, played a central part in facial makeup. The earliest evidence of the use of eye makeup comes from graves of the Badarian period (c. 4000 BCE), in which makeup substances and palettes for grinding them have been found. Painting the eyes, besides being part of magico-religious ritual, also had medical purposes – as protection against eye diseases. The eye-paint repelled the little flies that transmitted eye inflammations, prevented the delicate skin around the eyes from drying, and sheltered the eyes from the glare of the desert sun. And when Egyptian women realized that the painted frame also added emphasis to the eyes and made them appear larger, they began using eye makeup to enhance their beauty.

From the numerous surviving representations of Egyptian women of the ancient times we learn that they used to paint the upper eyelids and the eyebrows black and the lower line of the eye green. The black paint was made from galena, and the green from malachite. Malachite was used from the Pre-dynastic period onwards until at least the XIXth Dynasty, while the use of galena began afterwards. In later periods, Egyptian women made up their eyes with kohl prepared from sunflower soot, charred almond shells, and frankincense, and this practice is still prevalent in some parts of the world. Galena and malachite have been found in tombs, having been brought there as funerary gifts, frequently inside bags made of leather or linen. Quite often, beside the makeup materials, grinding palettes have been found as well – some simple and others designed in geometric forms or animal shapes – and these probably served to grind the makeup materials into a powder.

The powdered minerals were mixed with water, sometimes with the addition of a resin, and the preparation was kept in shells. In the course of time, the Egyptians began producing special containers for the kohl – the common name for eye-paint – in a wide variety of forms and materials. Some kohl containers have been found together with small sticks, stuck into them or tied to their necks. These little sticks, thickened at one end and flat at the other, were made of ivory, bone, wood, hematite, glass, or bronze. They were used for mixing the material, for extracting some of it from the container, and for applying

Woman coloring her cheeks in front of a mirror, Egypt

it around the eyes. The women would dip these sticks into water or perfumed oil and then into the makeup material, and in this way paint the eyes. The numerous kohl containers found attest to the widespread use of eye paint among the ancient Egyptians.

Apart from painting their eyes, Egyptian women also rouged their lips and cheeks. The main evidence that women colored their lips comes from the Turin "Erotic Papyrus," from the New Kingdom, in which a woman is depicted holding a mirror in one hand and making up her lips with the other, apparently with a brush. We also know that it was customary to color the face dark red with hematite and red ochre, which were mixed with vegetable oil or animal fat – both materials that have been found in numerous tombs. The Babylonians too used red ochre for facial makeup, but the Sumerians preferred yellow ochre. Herodotus, writing in the 5th century BCE, relates that the Babylonians painted their faces with vermilion and white lead and their eyes with kohl (*gukhlu*). Scholars assume that the kohl of the Babylonians was composed of natural arsenic, a white metallic material which turns black on exposure to air.

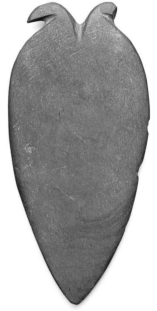

Palette for grinding makeup materials, slate, Egypt, Pre-dynastic period

While the purpose of makeup paints was to embellish the face and to emphasize its features, the ointments were used to soften and protect the skin, to preserve its freshness and rejuvenate its appearance. The hot and dry climatic conditions of Egypt made it necessary to take measures to prevent the skin from drying and wrinkling. The ointments were prepared from vegetable oils and sometimes from animal fat, and at times aromatic resin or perfumed beeswax were added. For the mixing of the solid components of the ointments, milk and honey were used. A papyrus from the 16th century BCE contains detailed recipes for ointments to remove blemishes, wrinkles, and other signs of age. For the removal of wrinkles, for example, it is recommended to prepare an ointment from a mixture of gum of frankincense, wax, fresh oil, and cypress kernels, pounded and mixed with milk, and to apply this preparation to the face for six days. Generally, these ointments have not been preserved, but in the tomb of the three princesses of the XVIIIth Dynasty in Thebes, jars were found with residual sediments. Analysis of the sediments has identified a mixture of a fat of some kind with lime or chalk. It would seem that this substance was used to cleanse the face.

Egyptian women kept their ointment jars, razors, mirrors and sometimes also their jewelry in special boxes, which were often exquisitely beautiful ornamental objects. The boxes, mostly rectangular, were made of wood inlaid with bone, ivory, or other materials, and in special cases were decorated with gold or silver frames. The boxes were subdivided into compartments, and some even had drawers for particular objects. At first the compartments were made to contain seven alabaster jars; in the course of time an eighth jar was added. The box was closed by simple means, mostly by tying a cord around knobs on the box and the lid. A woman who could not afford an elegant wooden box kept her ointments and other personal treasures in baskets made of rushes or straw. The Egyptian lady mostly stored the box under her bed, and at times it is depicted placed beside her chair.

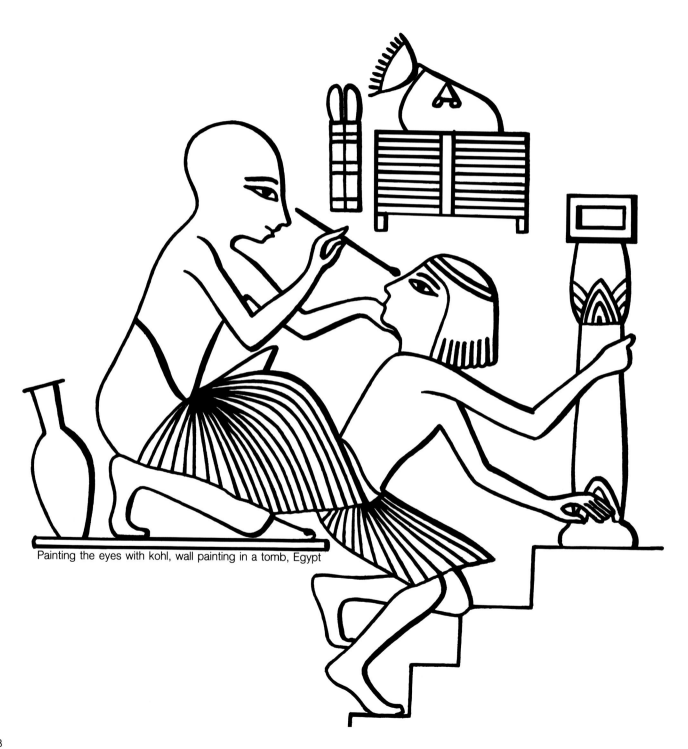

Painting the eyes with kohl, wall painting in a tomb, Egypt

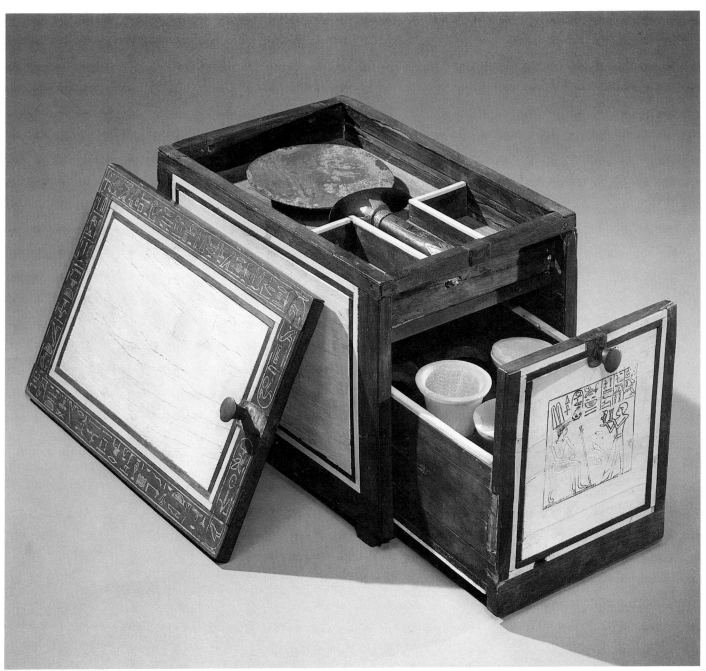

Toilet box, wood inlaid with ebony and ivory, Egypt, early 18th century BCE

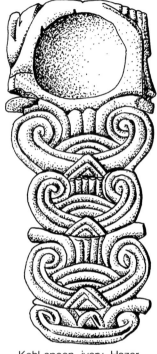

Kohl spoon, ivory, Hazor,
first half of 8th century BCE

Of the makeup practices among Hebrew women during the biblical period we have almost no knowledge, mainly becasue of the absence of pictorial or plastic representations, such as paintings and statues, in Eretz Israel. Though some figurines of the Astarte type from the First Temple period have been found with traces of paint visible on their faces, this is hardly sufficient to provide a clear idea of the makeup practices of the time. Nevertheless, we have no doubt that making up the face was customary in Israel, mainly because of the many implements and accessories found in excavations whose shape attests that they were used for makeup. These objects include popular utensils, such as stone cosmetic palettes which were common in the First Temple period (see below), as well as luxury items, such as the ivory kohl spoon found in one of the houses at Hazor, dating from the first half of the 8th century BCE. The handle of the spoon is carved with inverted palmettes and the back with a female head, flanked by doves. Another ivory box from Hazor, which dates from the same period, is decorated with a "Tree of Life" design flanked by a kneeling man and a sphinx; apparently it had served to contain an expensive ointment. Similar ivory items have been found in Mesopotamia.

The use of kohl for painting the eyes is mentioned three times in the Bible, always with disapprobation. When Jezebel, the wife of king Ahab, heard of the imminent arrival of Jehu, "she painted her eyes" (2 Kings, 9:30). Jeremiah, comparing Jerusalem to a harlot embellishing herself, uses the expression "you enlarge your eyes with paint" (4:30), and Ezekiel uses a similar figure of speech (23:40). In contrast, Job named one of his daughters "Keren Happukh" – "horn of eye-paint" (Job, 42:14).

As against the meager variety of makeup implements and the disapproval of such practices in sources of the First Temple period, there is widespread evidence of facial care and treatment from the Second Temple period. By now makeup was considered part of a woman's adornment: "These are permitted in a woman's adornments: she treats her eyes with kohl, fixes a parting and puts rouge on her face" (Babyl. *Moed Kattan*, 9b).

Jewish sources distinguish between makeup used for therapeutic purposes and makeup meant for embellishing the eyes: "Kohl, Rabbi Shema ben Elazar says, if for healing to kohl one eye, and if for ornament to kohl both eyes" (Tosefta *Shabbath*, 8:33). Elsewhere it is said that the "kohl (stibium) . . . stops the tears and promotes the growth of the eyelashes" (Babyl. *Shabbath*, 109a). Since making up the eyes was considered a labor, it was forbidden on the Sabbath: "She who paints is culpable on the score of dyeing" (Babyl. *Shabbath*, 95a); and during mourning the husband must exempt the wife from using makeup (Babyl. *Moed Kattan*, 20b).

The kohl stick and the kohl container were both used for painting the eyes and they are mentioned together in the Mishnah: "Sheath for the brush and receptacle for the eye-paint" (*Kelim*, 16:8). The kohl container characteristic of this period was a long, narrow glass tube, and multiple containers consisting of two to four tubes, presumably for differ-

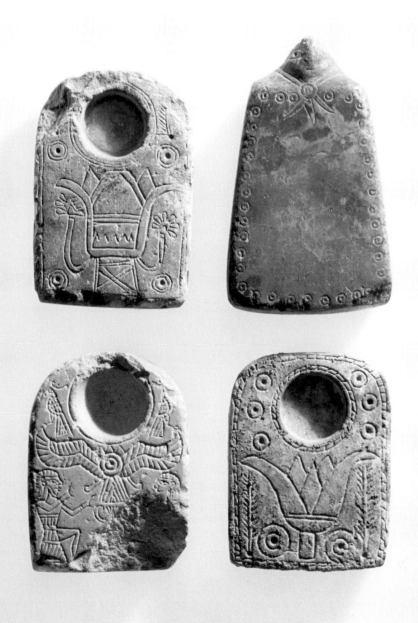

Palettes of Phoenician type for mixing cosmetics, limestone and alabaster, 8th–7th centuries BCE

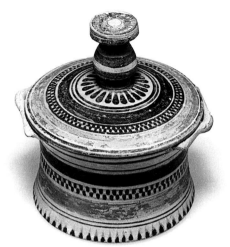

Pyxis (box) for cosmetics, pottery, Greece, 7th century BCE

ent colors. Many of these containers are decorated with glass threads and have basket handles for hanging. The Talmud tells of a woman who wished to be buried with her comb and her tube of eye-paint (Babyl. *Berakhot*, 18b). The tube mentioned probably refers to the commonly used glass tubes described above.

Often the container is found with the kohl stick inside it. This stick, usually made of bronze, was thickened at one end, for applying the paint – the "male" end, in the language of the Mishnah – while the other, the "female" end, was shaped like a little spoon or spatula, used to extract the paint from the container: "A kohl stick that has lost its ear spoon it is still susceptible (to uncleanness) because of its point (the male part); if it has lost its point, it is still susceptible because of its ear-spoon" (Mishnah *Kelim*, 13:2).

Applying makeup to the cheeks is also mentioned in the sources, and it too is forbidden on the Sabbath (Mishnah *Shabbath*, 10:6). It was customary to put light red or mauve makeup on the cheeks, and it is possible that a white powder was used as well. There is also mention of a white cosmetic powder made of flour, of which it is said that it must be removed from the house before the Passover with all the other items containing leavened flour (Mishnah *Pesahim*, 3:1).

In Greece and Rome, facial treatment was very highly developed and women devoted many hours to it. They used to spread various creams on the face and to apply makeup in vivid and contrasting colors. Greek women would cover their faces in the evening with a "beauty mask" that consisted mainly of flour, leaving it on their face all night. The next morning they would wash it off with milk. This mask was intended to remove blemishes from the skin and to endow it with a smooth and fresh appearance, ready for makeup. Dioscorides lists several recipes for preparing facial masks from various mixtures of honey, egg-white, bread crumbs or dough. A detailed description of a facial mask has reached us from testimonies about Poppaea, the wife of Nero, who was renowned for her ostentation. She used to wash off her facial mask in the morning with asses' milk, before making up her face.

During the classical period, a well-born girl would endeavor to make her skin look as light or as rosy as possible. Hence faces were made up with a white lead powder, even though people already knew about the harmfulness of lead. In Athenian tombs of the 3rd century BCE, white lead has been found. The lips and cheeks were generally painted a bright red. For certain colors the ancient Greeks used extracts of vegetables, seaweed, and mulberry fucus (a lichen). The eyes and eyebrows were painted black, with antimony (a crystalline metallic element) or with soot. The makeup fashionable among Greek women evokes a garish and to our taste certainly vulgar picture, but contemporary authors too expressed criticism of women who were made up in "a cheap and coarse" manner (Xenophon, *Oeconomicus*, X:2), because already in those times, exaggerated and heavy makeup was characteristic of prostitutes.

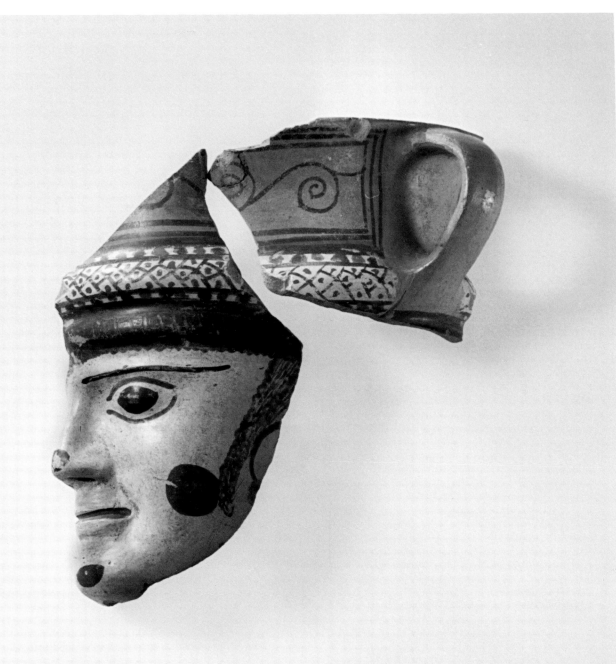

Vase in the shape of a human head with painted face, terra-cotta, West Anatolia, c. mid-5th century BCE

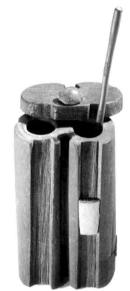

Double kohl tube and stick,
wood, Egypt, New Kingdom

The Romans at first used few cosmetics, but with the influx of Greek customs the practice of making up the face spread quickly, among both men and women. The Roman lady had a special maidservant who was responsible for all cosmetic matters: the *ornatrix*. The Roman style of makeup was similar to the Greek, and the lightening of facial color was achieved not only with white lead but also with white excrements of crocodiles. The makeup materials and ointments were kept in handsome containers and were sometimes placed in a special box.

The great importance attached to cosmetics in the classical world also found expression in the extensive literature on the subject, including recipes for makeup preparations. Queen Cleopatra VII, who lived in the mid-1st century BCE is said to have written a famous book on beautification. The book itself has not survived, but it is extensively quoted by various authors from the Roman period and even later.

The kohl and powder containers and the various ointment boxes were remarkable for their fine designs and for the costly materials from which they were made. Especially renowned for their skill in this industry were the Egyptians, and the Greeks too produced containers that were traded in the entire Mediterranean basin. Many of the Egyptian cosmetic containers were made of stone, mainly because stone has the virtue of preserving low temperatures and keeping the contents fresh. In Greece, however, most of the containers were made of pottery, and these are remarkable for their exquisite paintings, which depict uses of cosmetics. A selection of the implements and containers used for facial treatment in various areas and periods is illustrated here.

The typical Egyptian kohl container in use during the Middle Kingdom was a squat alabaster pot with a flat bottom, wide rim, and narrow mouth. This pot was equipped with a flat lid, and it was occasionally mounted on a small, four-legged stand. With slight changes in form, this type of pot continued to be popular also in the New Kingdom. It often bears labels such as: "Good for the sight," "To stanch bleeding," "To cause tears," etc. Kohl tubes – often double tubes – made of bone, ivory, or faience, were also used in Egypt during this period. These too bore labels indicating their purpose: "For daily use," a powder "For cleaning the eyes," and the like. Multiple kohl containers made of four tubes, each of which contained a different color, for each season of the year, are also known. Most distinctive are the kohl containers designed in the shape of a woman or a monkey, squatting or standing and holding a container. Numerous containers like these, made of stone, wood, and other materials have been found. A stone container of this type has also been unearthed in Palestine, in a burial cave at Gezer, dating from c. 1400 BCE; this specimen consists of two containers shaped like monkeys standing on their hind legs and holding a basket. Another type of kohl container, which first appears in the New Kingdom, is made of polychrome glass in the shape of a palm.

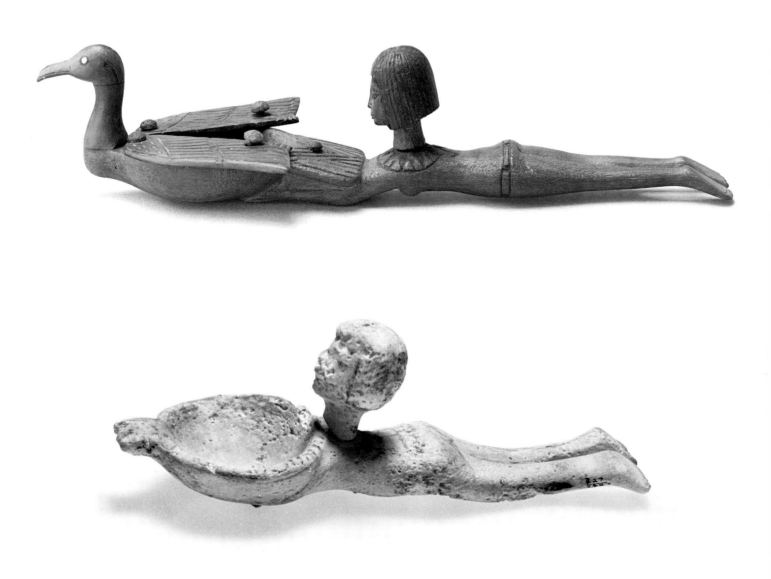

Cosmetic spoons in the shape of swimming girls.
Top: wood and ivory, Egypt, XVIIIth Dynasty; bottom: alabaster, Deir el-Balah, 13th century BCE

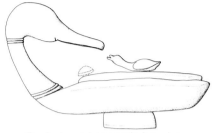

Duck-shaped cosmetic box, ivory,
Akko, 14th–13th centuries BCE

Animal-shaped kohl containers were prevalent in Afghanistan at the beginning of the 2nd millennium BCE. Some of these feature a realistic design with close attention to detail, while others are schematically fashioned. In some cases, the container's opening is in the head of the figure, and in others a tube extends upwards from the back of the animal and serves as an opening. At times the container is equipped with a loop to which the kohl stick is attached with a chain. In the same period, small, heart-shaped metal bottles with a high neck were produced in the Indus valley, as well as square stone bottles with a short cylindrical neck, and decorated by geometric designs on the sides. It is likely that these too served as kohl containers.

Around the middle of the 1st millennium BCE (6th–4th centuries BCE), kohl containers of colored glass were produced in a variety of shapes – square, cylindrical, pear- or heart-shaped – and these apparently originated from Northwest Iran. The body of these containers was sometimes decorated with colored glass threads in various designs, and sometimes with knobs on the shoulder.

The Egyptians also excelled in the manufacture of tiny containers for ointments and cosmetic powders, and they have left us a wide variety of these exquisite vessels. Among them are many squat containers made of stone or alabaster. These Egyptian containers also reached Palestine, and beautiful specimens have been found in the treasury of the Late Canaanite palace at Megiddo (Stratum VIII). Especially handsome are the cosmetic spoons designed in the shape of swimming girls. Such spoons, made of ivory or wood, have been found in Egypt, Palestine, Syria, and Cyprus. They were especially popular in the New Kingdom. Their handles take the shape of a young maiden whose legs extend backwards and whose arms stretch forward clasping a container, which may be round, rectangular, or shaped like a fish or duck. At times the container has a lid attached by a hinge. The girl, whose hair is arranged in an elaborate Egyptian style, is practically nude but for a collar and a girdle. An alabaster spoon of this type, dating from the 13th century BCE, has been found at Deir el-Balah, and several ivory spoons like these have been uncovered at Megiddo. Although these spoons are believed by many scholars to have served as cosmetic utensils, their function is not certain, since no depictions of such spoons in an appropriate context are known. Their small size, however, shows that they had contained some precious substance.

Spoons of another kind, elegant and delicate in their design, were common in the New Kingdom, and these too are generally seen as perfume or cosmetic spoons. They are made of alabaster, bone, or wood, and their handles are designed in the shape of a human figure or decorated with plant motifs. Occasionally the entire spoon is shaped like an animal, such as an ibex or an oryx, with its feet bound. The exact purpose of these spoons is also uncertain, and almost no traces of materials remain on them for analysis, except for one spoon in the British Museum, which was examined at the beginning of the present century and found to have contained an oily substance.

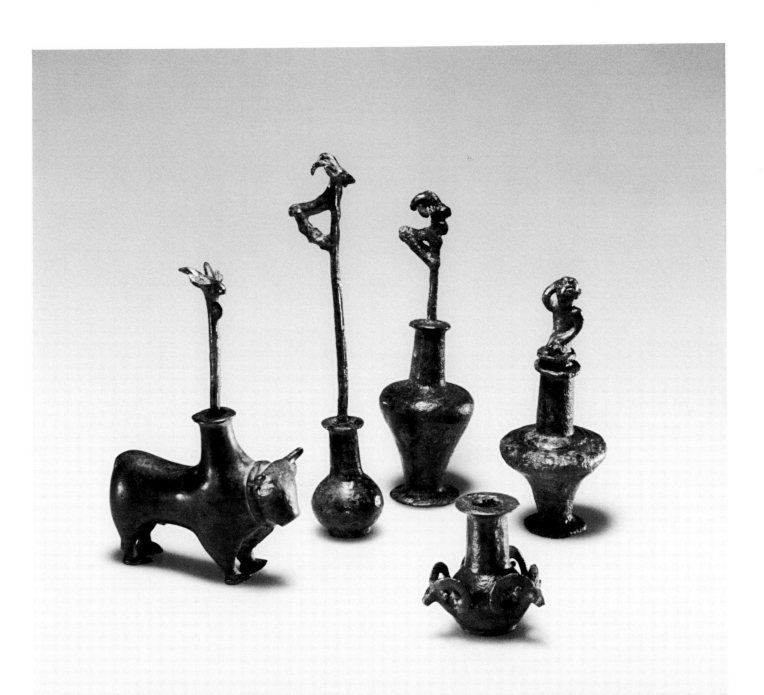

Kohl containers and kohl sticks, bronze, Afghanistan, early 2nd millennium BCE

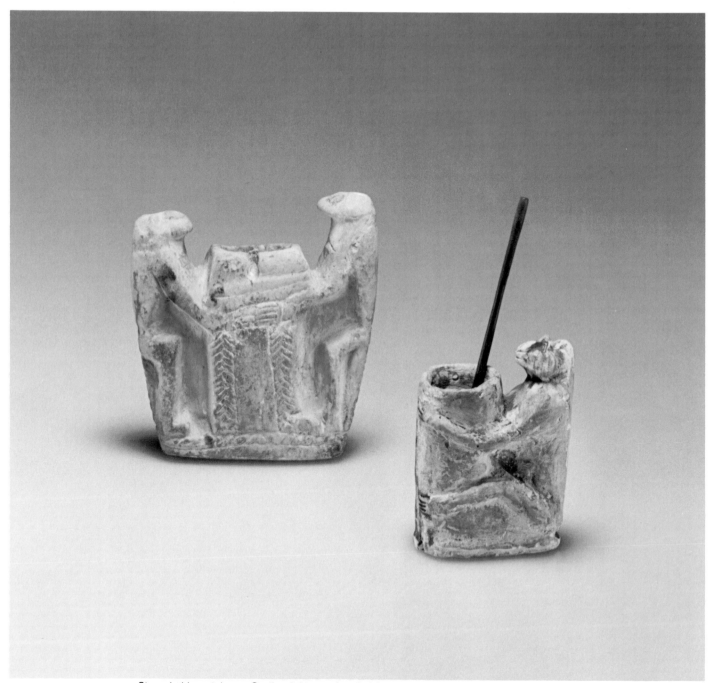

Stone kohl containers. On the right: monkey holding a container, Egypt, New Kingdom;
on the left: pair of monkeys clasping a basket, Gezer, c. 1400 BCE

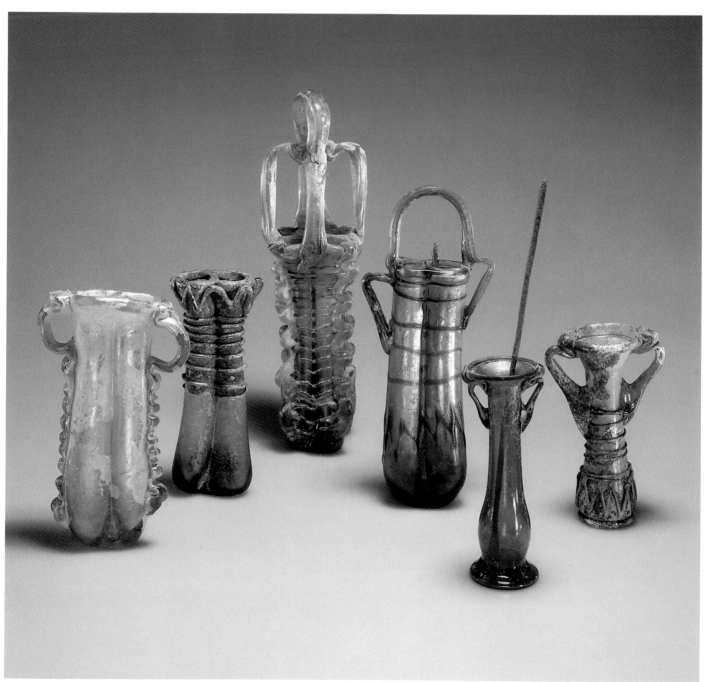

Multiple kohl tubes, glass (some contained a bronze kohl stick), Eretz Israel, 3rd–5th centuries CE

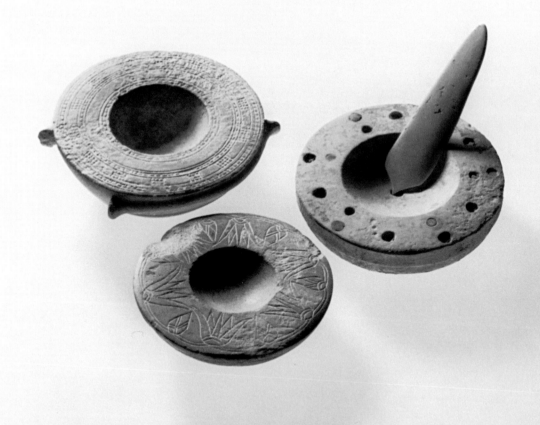

Decorated bowls for grinding and mixing cosmetics, stone, Eretz Israel, 8th–7th centuries BCE

The majority of these spoons have been unearthed from tombs of men, women, and children, sometimes beside cosmetic implements, and only a few have been found in houses or palaces. Another source of such spoons are temples, suggesting that they were used ritually for incense-burning, although no traces of soot have remained on them. It has also been suggested that the spoons designed in the shapes of bound animals symbolized a sacrifice. It is therefore reasonable to assume that these spoons were used for both womens' cosmetics and ritual practices, in view of the fact that statues of the gods received daily cosmetic treatment. The presence of such spoons in tombs may perhaps be connected to rituals of washing the dead and the statues of the dead.

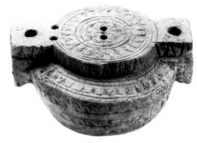

Pyxis (box) for cosmetics, ivory, Tel Dan, 14th century BCE

In the second half of the 2nd millennium BCE, duck-shaped cosmetic boxes also became popular along the Syro-Palestinian coast and in the Aegean world. In our region, these have been found at Megiddo, Dan, Gezer, Lachish, Sidon, Ugarit, Alalakh, and Hamid el-Loz. They are mostly made of hippopotamus ivory, and the heads of the ducks are generally turned backwards. The lids, attached by hinges, consist of a pair of wings or of a single piece, sometimes with ducklings sitting on top, so that the mother-duck turns her head towards her offspring. Boxes of this type, made of ivory and wood, are also known from Egypt, but since their main distribution area is along the Syro-Palestinian coast, their origin should probably be traced to the Syro-Canaanite world.

Among the cosmetic utensils used for making up the eyes or face one must include the stone bowls which were widespread in Eretz Israel, Transjordan and Phoenicia in the 8th–7th centuries BCE. These are cosmetic palettes with a round hollow at the center for grinding the material or mixing it with oil to make it easy to spread. Next to such a palette, excavated at Hazor, a small pestle has been found that fits the hollow in the palettes. The palettes are well polished inside and outside and are usually decorated on their rims with simple geometric designs. Exceptional among these bowls is a palette decorated with a lotus design; other outstanding examples are inlaid with glass, reminiscent of ivories inlaid in various colors. A few palettes of glass, faience, and ivory, which imitate the stone palettes, have also been found.

Another kind of utensil for grinding cosmetic substances are palettes made of alabaster or limestone, dating from the 7th century BCE. These palettes are designed in the shape of a schematically represented female figure, with a carved head at the top and circles at the edges which may represent the hem of her garment. One of these palettes has a carved figure with a distinctive hairdo consisting of four braids crowned with a diadem, and holding a lotus blossom. Another palette has a female figure wearing a chain around her neck, with a pomegranate-shaped medallion hanging from it. These palettes are reminiscent of the heads decorating *tridacna* shells (see below).

Also from this period are elongated stone palettes featuring a rounded upper part with a hollow similar to the one in the cosmetic palettes. On one of these palettes a cult scene

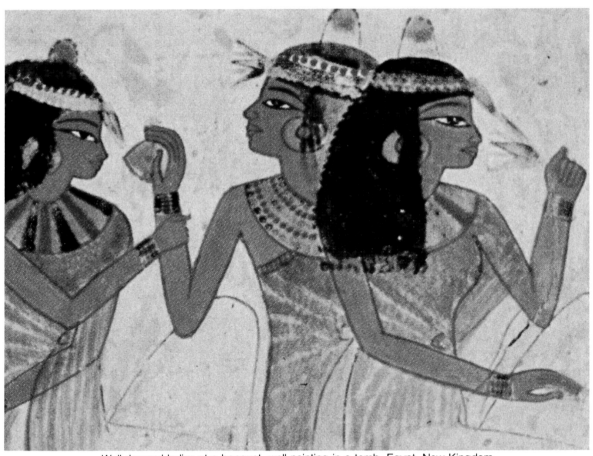

Well-dressed ladies at a banquet, wall painting in a tomb, Egypt, New Kingdom

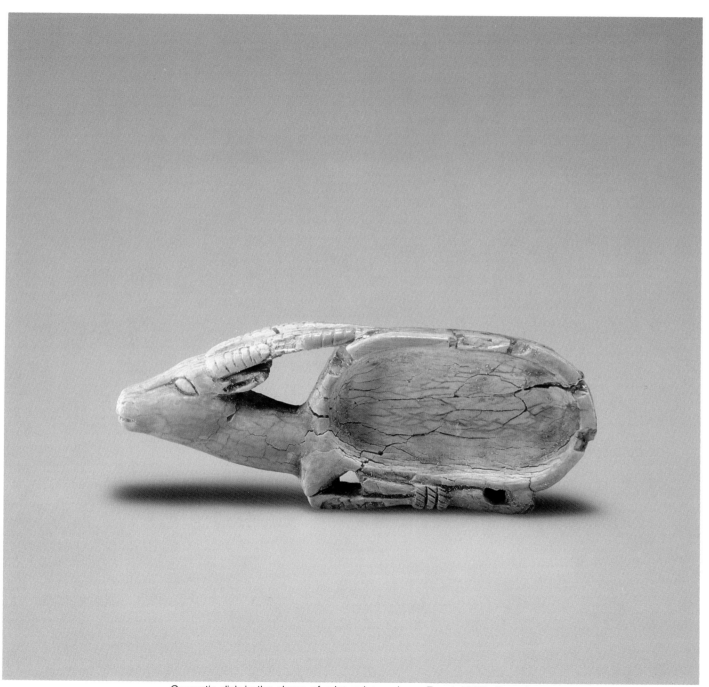

Cosmetic dish in the shape of a bound oryx, ivory, Egypt, XVIIIth Dynasty

is engraved, depicting the "Tree of Life," surmounted by a winged disk and flanked by kneeling figures with hands raised in prayer or blessing. Another palette is decorated with a lotus blossom at the center, and a palmette on either side. Yet another has an engraving of a stylized lotus blossom, with two stems rising from it and a flower at the top. These motifs come from the world of Phoenician art and are reminiscent of the designs encountered on the ivories.

Two cosmetic vessels from this period should be mentioned here, one from Hazor and the other from Samaria. The Hazor goblet is crudely made and decorated with a geomet-

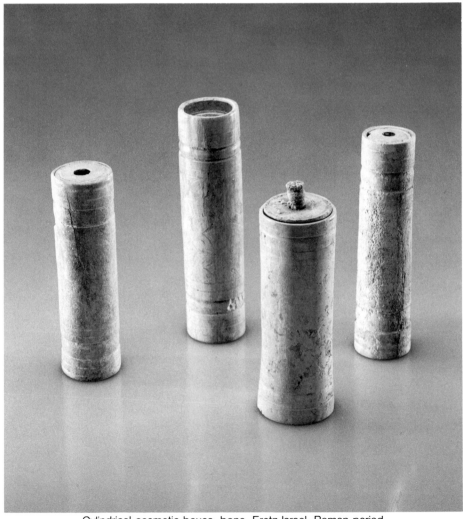

Cylindrical cosmetic boxes, bone, Eretz Israel, Roman period

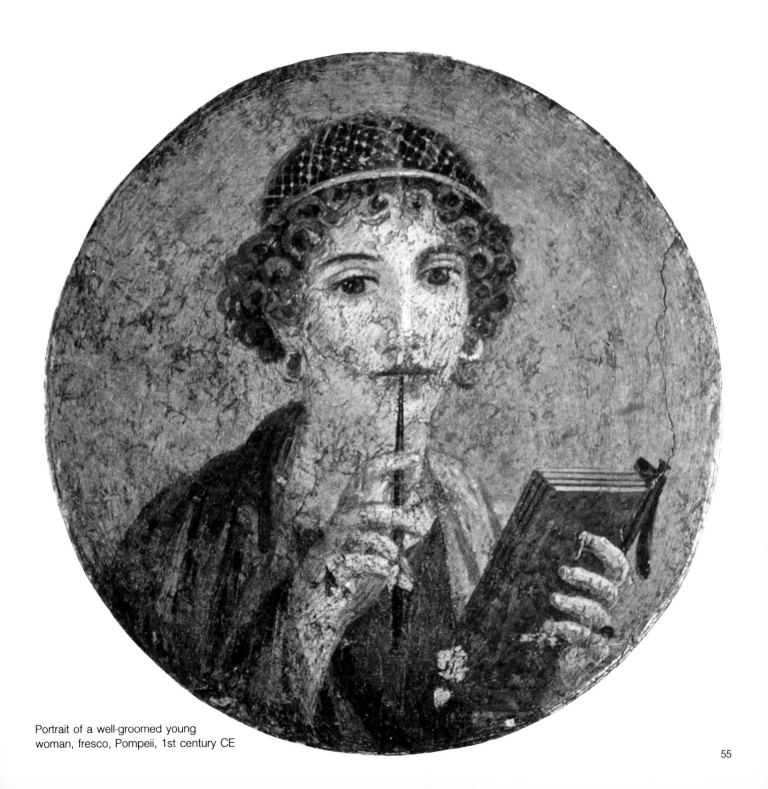

Portrait of a well-groomed young
woman, fresco, Pompeii, 1st century CE

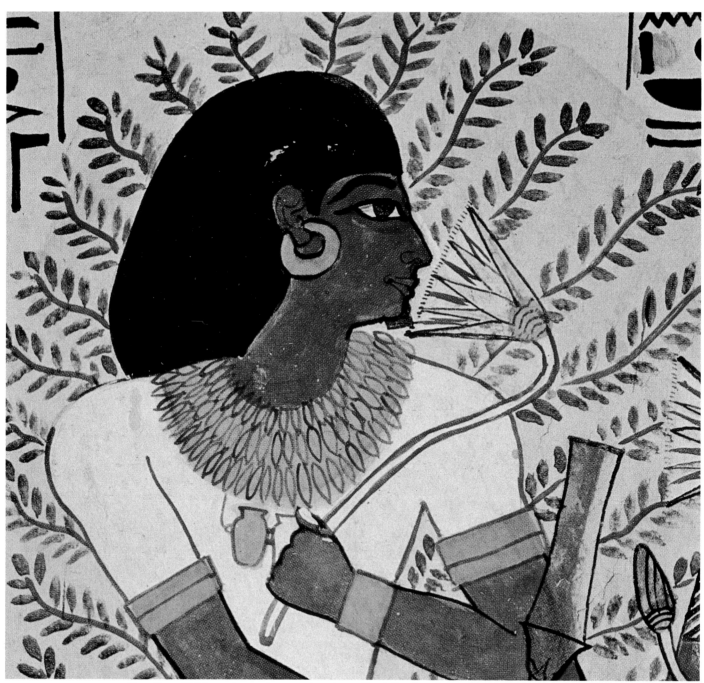

Egyptian official wearing makeup and a wig, wall painting in a tomb, Egypt, New Kingdom

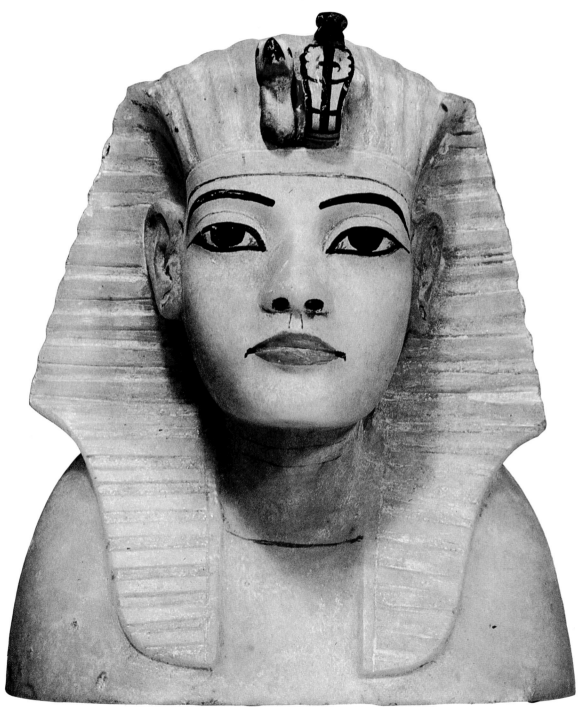

Regal portrait of Tut-Ankh-Amon, alabaster, Egypt, New Kingdom

ric pattern similar to that on the cosmetic palettes. This goblet originally had a lid, which has not survived. The goblet from Samaria, remarkably beautiful, is made in the shape of a flower with six sepals and ten petals.

Yet another group of cosmetic containers is made of *tridacna* shells (*Tridacna Squamosa*). A number of studies have shown that since the earliest times shells have been used as containers for cosmetics, and both the ground and the mixed substances were kept in them. The distinction of the *tridacna* shell lies in its exquisite decorations. These shells, which became popular during the 7th century BCE, mainly in the eastern part of the Mediterranean basin, had decorations on the outside and also a narrow strip of decoration on the inside. Usually the decorations depict a winged figure wearing a robe ornamented with squares, whose head, as already noted, recalls the female heads carved on the stone palettes. The decorated *tridacna* shells, which were undoubtedly luxury items, have mostly been found in private homes, and would seem to have been in everyday use. The shell illustrated here was discovered in the courtyard of the citadel at Arad, and has been dated to the second half of the 7th century BCE.

Of special interest among the cosmetic containers from the Hellenistic period are tiny pottery vessels, some bearing names, which were also prevalent in Palestine. These are generally thought to have been containers for cosmetic ointments, and it has recently been suggested that the ointments in question were medicinal and that the name engraved on them designated the name of the ointment, or of the pharmacist. But the distinction between medicinal and cosmetic uses was quite vague, then as now.

In the Roman period another kind of container was also in use in Palestine – a cylindrical, lidded box, made of pottery, glass, or bone, in which cosmetic powders or ointments were kept. A rare example of such containers is the wooden box that was preserved in the Cave of Letters in the Judaean Desert, albeit without any trace of its contents. In various places in the Greek and Roman world boxes with lids (pyxides), containing rouge and other makeup materials, have been found. Boxes such as these are depicted in vase paintings and on tombstones as being part of a woman's equipment. Flat and round boxes of bronze and marble were also used for the same purpose.

Interestingly enough, in Greece and Rome we find none of the special kohl containers which were so popular in the East. It would seem that for these purposes ordinary narrow and cylindrical receptacles were used.

It appears, then, that although the various materials used for makeup during ancient times changed in composition, and the cosmetic containers sometimes changed their form, people's concept of beauty and their urge to beautify themselves have remained virtually unchanged from time immemorial.

# Hair and Hair-styles

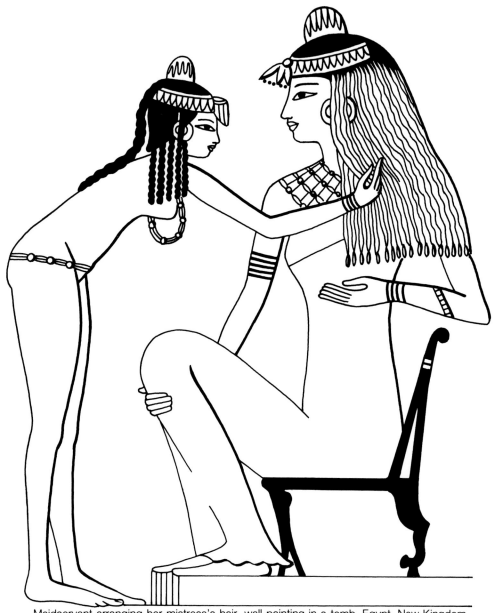

Maidservant arranging her mistress's hair, wall painting in a tomb, Egypt, New Kingdom

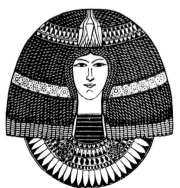

Elaborate stylized wig of an Egyptian lady, detail from a painting on a sarcophagus

The hair-styles known to us from antiquity are many and varied, and reflect the changing fashions among different peoples during different periods. From them we can learn about the character of the period, but also about the status of the person. Our chief sources of information about hair-styles of the ancient world are sculptures, reliefs, wall paintings, and coins.

In prehistoric periods the hair and beard were allowed to grow wild. It was only from the 3rd millennium BCE on that people began to be conscious about their appearance, and attempted to improve it. Among other things, men now began to cut their hair and shave their beards. Hair was a symbol of strength, and a person whose hair was shorn regarded that as a loss of his strength, as in the words of Samson: "If I be shaven, then my strength will leave me" (Judges, 16:17). Grasping a man by the hair was taken as an act of subjugation, as seen in ancient Egyptian depictions where the king is shown grasping his enemy by the forelock.

The Egyptians, who were very particular about body cleanliness, regarded long hair and a beard as a sign of neglect, and thus frequently shaved their beards as well as the hair of their head, or cropped the hair very short, as can be seen in their paintings and statues. Evidence of this custom is also found in the Bible: when Joseph was summoned to stand before Pharaoh, "they brought him hastily out of the dungeon, and he shaved himself and changed his clothes" (Genesis, 41:14). The Egyptian priests were required to pay particularly strict attention to cleanliness, and every three days they had to shave all their body hair, and even their eyebrows. However, instead of the natural hair wigs were worn and kings even wore artificial beards.

Egyptian wigs were short or long: the short wig was made of little overlapping curls arranged in horizontal rows which also covered most of the forehead; while the long wig, which was considered more elegant, flowed down to the shoulders and created a frame for the face. In Egyptian art, a bearded face and long hair generally identifies its wearer as a foreigner or a person from the lower classes.

Egyptian women generally wore their hair flowing down to the shoulders or even longer. During the Middle Kingdom they parted their hair in the middle, so that locks of hair reached down to the shoulders and the rest hung down their backs. This hair-style is characteristic of the Egyptian goddess Hathor. In New Kingdom art, women are shown wearing their hair long or plaited and falling to the shoulders. Many of these coiffures must have been wigs. It was customary to wear wigs on festive occasions, and it may be assumed that at least among the upper classes of the population, every man and woman owned a wig. In many cases wigs and locks of hair have been found among the funerary equipment in Egyptian tombs.

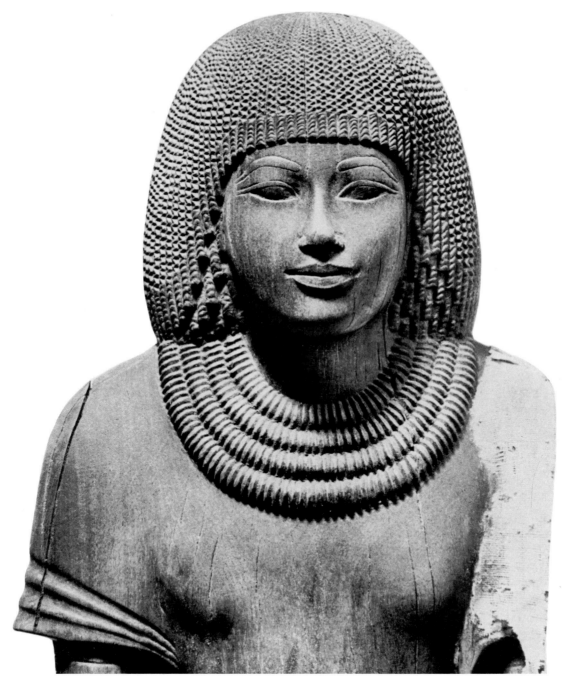

Portrait of an official wearing an elaborate wig, wood, Egypt, New Kingdom

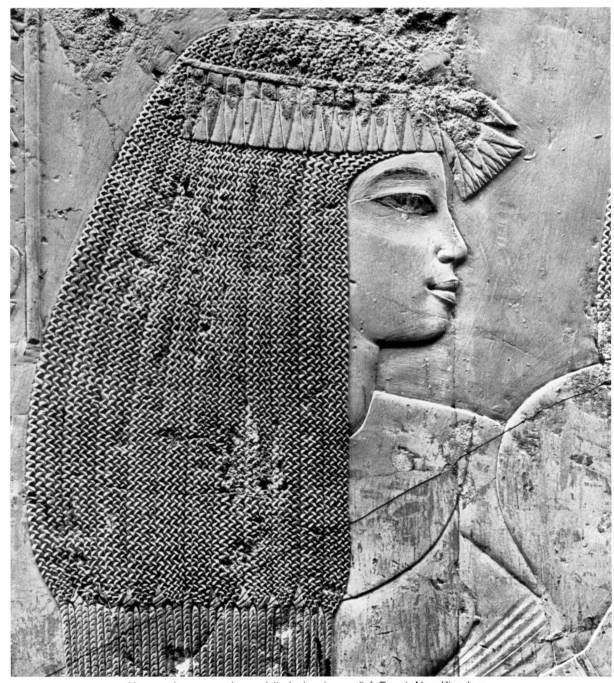

Young princess wearing a plaited wig, stone relief, Egypt, New Kingdom

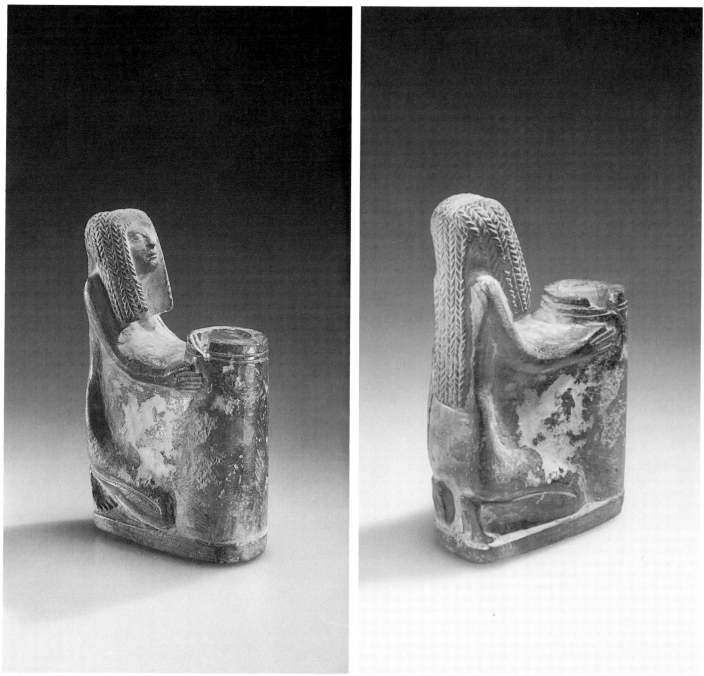

Kohl container in the shape of a woman wearing a long wig, stone, Egypt, New Kingdom

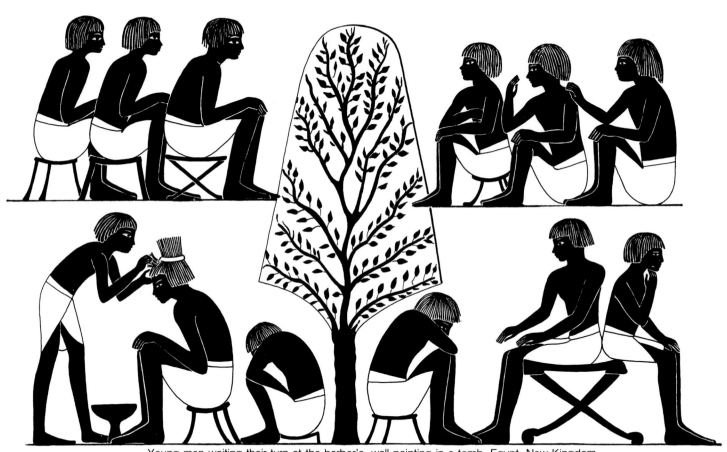

Young men waiting their turn at the barber's, wall painting in a tomb, Egypt, New Kingdom

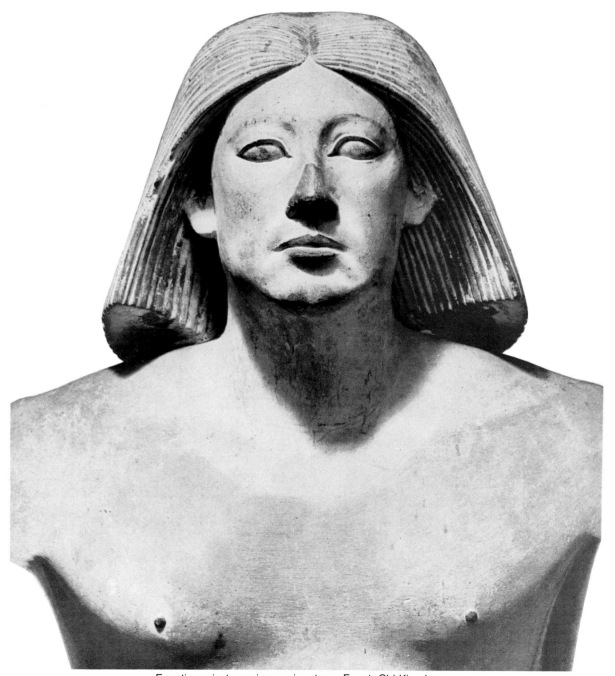

Egyptian priest wearing a wig, stone, Egypt, Old Kingdom

Arranging the curls of a wig, reconstruction

In depictions of banquets, a cone is shown on the heads of guests and even of servants. This cone was made of tallow impregnated with myrrh. It remained on the head throughout the banquet, and as time passed and the temperature rose the cone melted gradually into the hair and dripped down the face, releasing its fragrance. In wall paintings the cone is whitish, with orange-brown streaks which may represent the aromatic substance with which the fat was impregnated.

The wigs were mostly made of human hair and sometimes of horsehair, sheep's wool, or plant fibers. Some wigs were made of long, straight hair; others of short, curly hair. The hair in the wigs was dyed. Kings, for instance, wore green or blue wigs. Wigs have been found with traces of wax, which must have been used to hold the curls or the plaits in place. The complicated coiffures and wigs were designed by expert hairstylists, and at times one of the members of the family or one of the women of the harem arranged the hair of her mistress, as we can see from depictions on sarcophagi from the First Intermediate period. The relief on the sarcophagus of the Lady Kawit, of the Middle Kingdom, represents a hairdresser standing behind her mistress and arranging the hair of her curly wig, while the lady holds a mirror.

Men were shaved by a team of servants in the palace or the temple. But there were also barbers who served the general public. Few depictions showing a barber at his work have survived, and on these it is hard to distinguish his equipment. We can, however, see pails or ewers for water to wet the skin before shaving, and it seems likely that oil or unguents were used for softening the skin and the areas to be shaved. The shave was part of the daily routine of every man, who used his own personal implements, which included a metal razor, or a flint knife in earlier periods. The razor was kept in a special sheath made of bone or wood, or in a leather or linen bag or a basket, together with hairpins, combs, and other personal toilet gear.

One of the things that troubled the Egyptians who, as noted, greatly appreciated a well-groomed look, was the appearance of gray hair and baldness. Papyri have been discovered which record formulas for ointments to prevent hair loss. These ointments contained a mixture consisting of the fat of lion, hippopotamus, crocodile, cat, snake, and ibex. Thinning hair would be thickened by the addition of artificial hair, as we learn from the switches found in numerous tombs. To overcome the problem of graying hair, people treated it with a concoction that contained the blood of a black calf or a black bull, boiled in oil, in the belief that the color of the animal's hair would pass to the person using the mixture.

In Mesopotamia, in contrast to Egypt, during the Early Dynastic period men let their hair and beards grow. Depictions in art and literature show that there were different hair-styles for kings and for the common people. In Mesopotamia shaving was considered a mark of disgrace and also a sign of mourning. During periods of mourning the common people tore out their hair, and kings would shave their hair and fast in the face of imminent danger.

Hairdo of an Assyrian king, stone relief, 9th century BCE

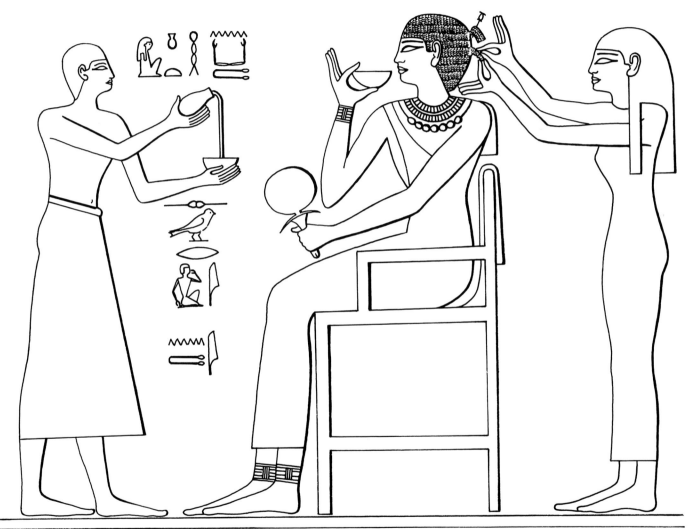

Egyptian lady having her hair dressed by a maidservant, relief on a sarcophagus, Egypt, Middle Kingdom

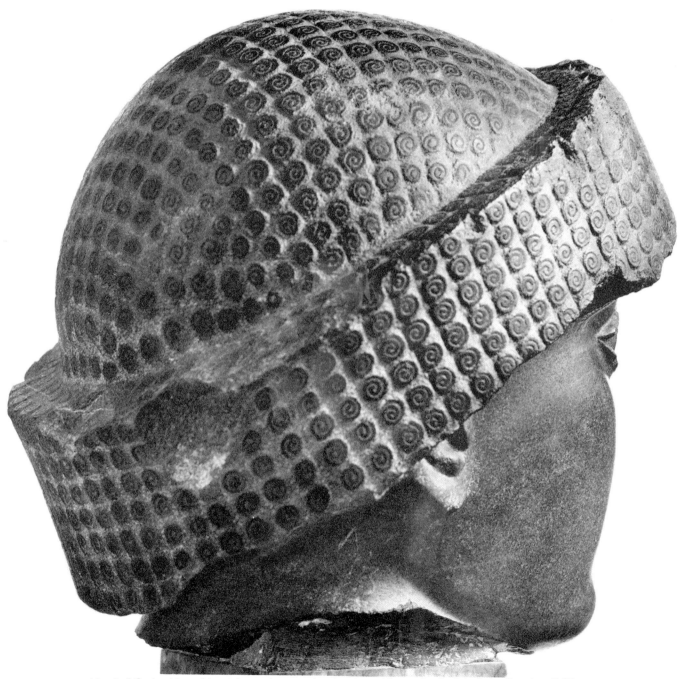

Head of Gudea king of Lagash wearing a curly wig, stone, Mesopotamia, late 3rd millennium BCE

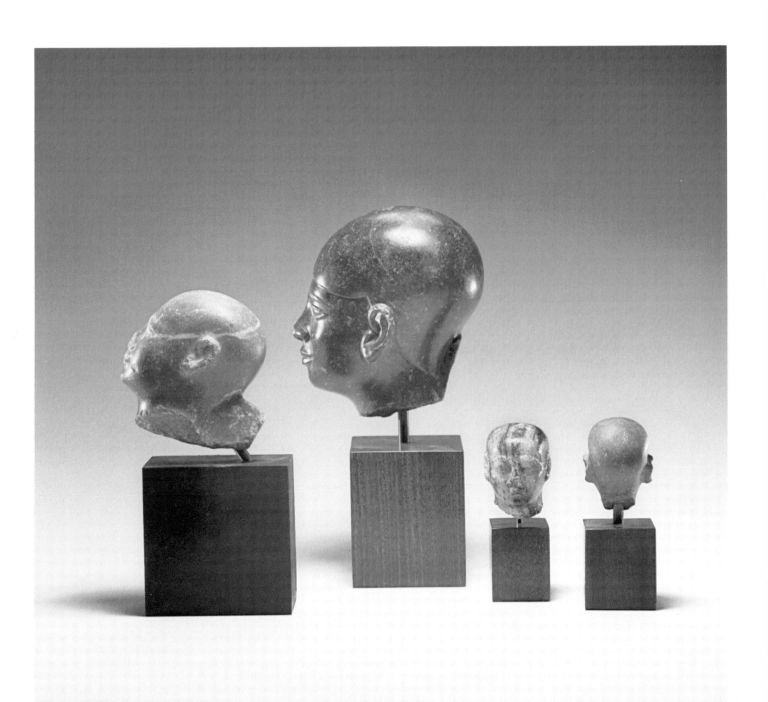

Bare-headed men, stone, Egypt, 2nd and 1st millennia BCE

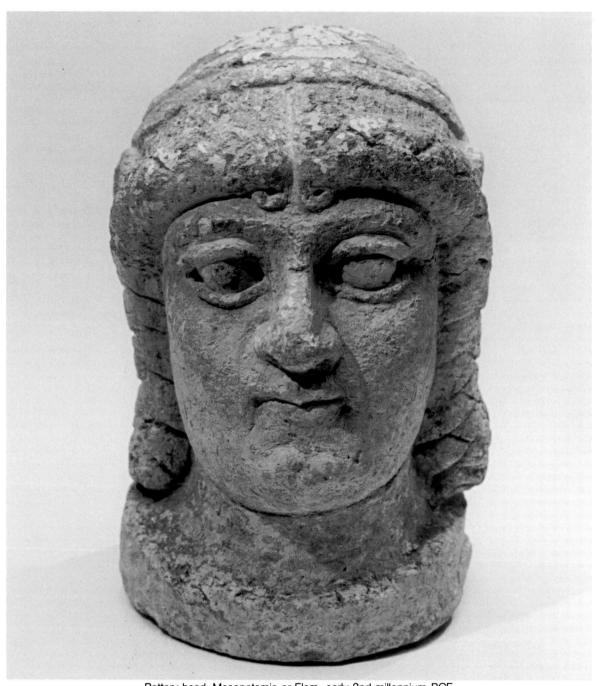

Pottery head, Mesopotamia or Elam, early 2nd millennium BCE

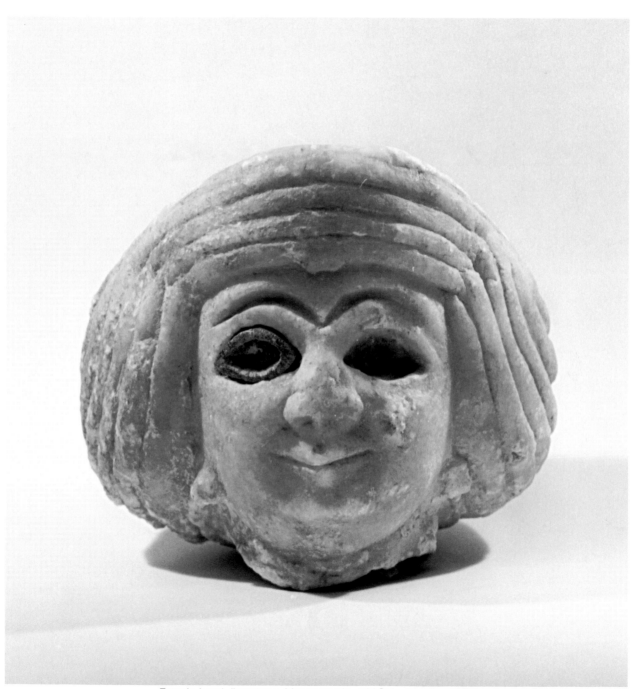

Female head, limestone, Mesopotamia, mid-3rd millennium BCE

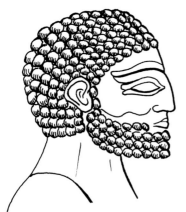

Hairdo of a Hebrew man,
detail from the Lachish reliefs,
late 8th century BCE

In the Neo-Sumerian period, on the other hand, men generally shaved their hair, as may be seen in the heads of the statues of Gudea, king of Lagash, from the late 3rd millennium BCE. However, the Sumerians also wore wigs and artificial beards, as in Egypt. The Sumerian women, in contrast, cherished their long hair and even made it look fuller with the aid of false hair or semi-wigs.

From the time of Hammurabi on, in the Early Babylonian period, men wore long beards. Towards the end of the 2nd millennium BCE, Assyrian kings began to be represented with long hair falling down the shoulders and curled at the ends, and with square beards made of groups of ringlets. Other men wore their hair shorter and also had shorter beards, which were always curled. The hair of the head and beard was usually covered with a thick layer of fat to prevent hair loss.

Women have always cherised long hair as an important part of their beauty. In Mesopotamian art women are sometimes seen with hair flowing down their backs in a thick plait or tied back with a ribbon. Sometimes they braided their hair into plaits which fell to the shoulders, or were wound around the head. During the Third Dynasty of Ur, in the late 3rd millennium BCE, it was the fashion to allow the hair to flow freely down the back and sometimes separate locks fell over the shoulders and chest. Assyrian women wore their hair shorter, braiding and binding it into a bun at the back of their heads. In the Neo-Babylonian period fashions changed and women wore curly fringes on their foreheads. The complicated hair-styles were arranged by professional hairdressers.

The hairdressers constituted an important and respected class in Mesopotamia, and were organized in a guild. In every town there were a number of hairdressers' shops, concentrated in a single street, which served the general public. In these shops the barbers would shave their clients – with a razor and pumice stone – and then massage them with unguents and perfumes. Barbers also performed medical functions such as treating slight wounds and shaving lepers so that they could be identified from afar.

The civilizations of Egypt and Mesopotamia have left us many plastic representations of hair-styles which were current in various periods and in different circles. As for the hair fashions of ancient Israel, however, we unfortunately have to rely almost entirely on written sources. Of the few artifacts which have come down to us, the plaques and figurines of fertility goddesses are of special importance in this respect. Their hair is usually arranged in an elaborate style, which evidently was characteristic of the wealthier women. Another source is the depiction on the Lachish reliefs, which show the inhabitants leaving the town and going into exile.

It appears that women in Israel generally grew their hair long and let it fall down to their shoulders, but some wore it gathered, or in plaits. Isaiah describes the hair-styles of the women of Jerusalem as "well-set hair" (3:24), meaning hair gathered and rolled into a knot

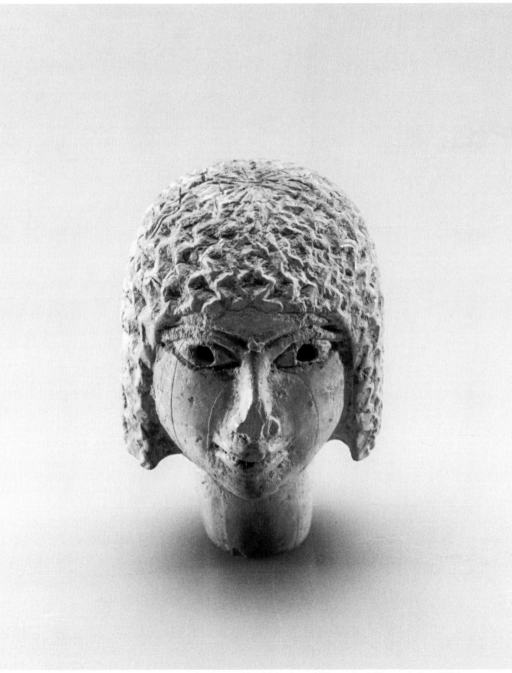

Head of a woman wearing a wig, ivory, Megiddo, late 13th–early 12th centuries BCE

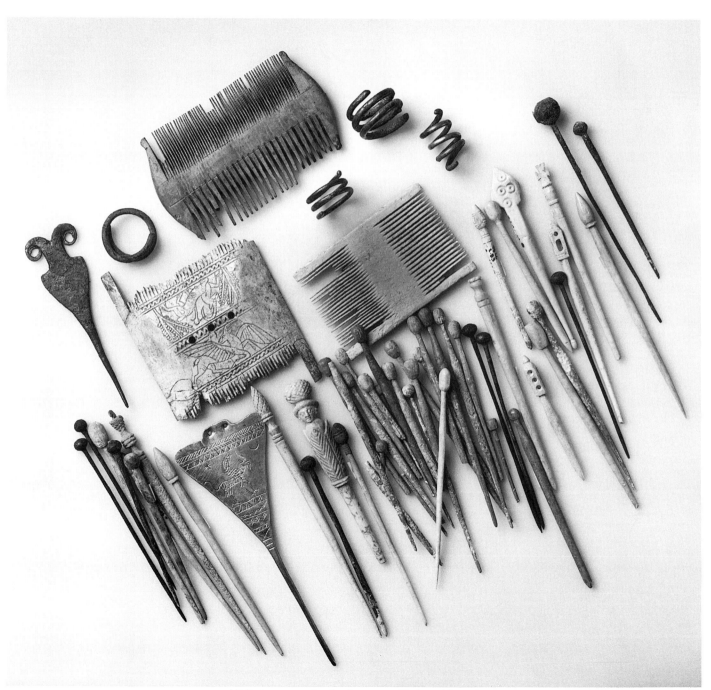

Various accessories for the care of hair and beard

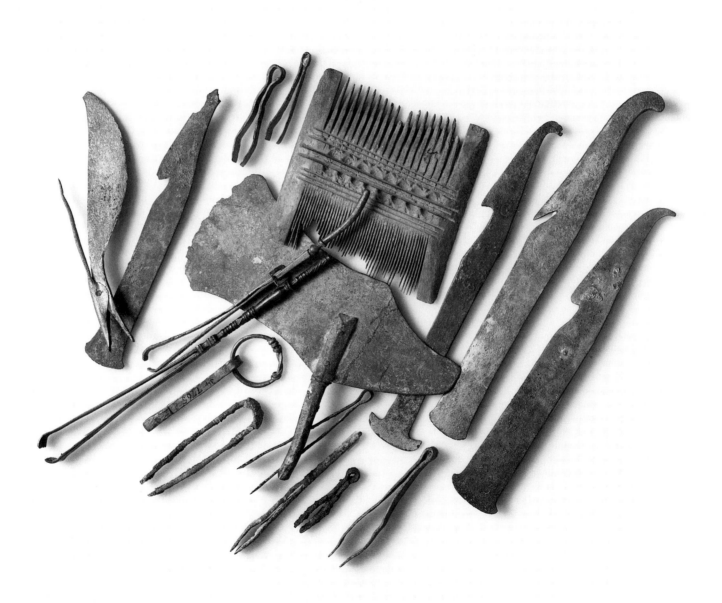

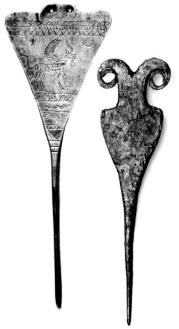

Hair-pins, silver and bronze,
Northwest Iran,
late 2nd–early 1st millennium BCE

at the back of the head, or a rolled-up plait held by a pin in the Mesopotamian style. A description of a beautiful woman with long hair is given in the Song of Solomon: "You are fair, my love . . . your hair is as a flock of goats, coming down from Mount Gilead" (4:1). Hair was also an important feature of male beauty: "His locks are bushy and black as a raven" (ibid., 5:11), and of Samson we are told that his hair was done in "seven locks" (Judges, 16:13).

In Israel the long and well-groomed beard was considered a mark of distinction: "It is like the precious oil upon the head running down upon the beard, upon the beard of Aaron that went down to the skirts of his garments" (Psalms, 133:2). The custom of shaving the beard and the hair of the head was not practiced by the Hebrews. The priests were forbidden to shave the hair of their heads and the edges of their beards (Leviticus, 21:5), and all Israelites were forbidden to cut their hair to an equal length, in a round shape, and also to shave the edges of their beards (Leviticus, 19:27). In the First Temple period, as we know from the Bible, a shaved head and beard was a sign of disgrace (2 Samuel, 10:4), and also of mourning (Jeremiah, 41:5), and it is upon this biblical injunction that the later prohibition against cutting the hair and shaving was established as one of the main precepts of mourning (Babyl. Moed Kattan, 14a).

In the period of the Mishnah and the Talmud, under the influence of Hellenistic culture, much attention was devoted to hair care among both men and women. The women's hair was mostly long – sometimes reaching down to the feet – but they did not allow it to flow free. It was braided into plaits and wound around the head, or gathered and fastened with ribbons, nets, clips or pins: "The needle which is unpierced . . . since a woman tidies her hair with it" (Babyl. Shabbath, 60a). A wealthy woman would have her private hairdresser (ibid., 94b), and ordinary women arranged their own hair. However, since the hair-style was sometimes elaborate and intricate, it was forbidden to unravel or arrange it on the Sabbath. Men too took regular care of their hair, and the higher a man's standing, the more often he visited the barber. Of Ben Elashah, son-in-law of Rabbi Judah the Prince, the Talmud writes: "Ben Elashah did not scatter his money in vain, but in order to show off the haircut in the style of the High Priest's haircut . . . like the Lulian style of haircutting . . . the style of a distinguished person" (Babyl. Nedarim, 51a). The Talmud set fixed times for hairdressing: the king will cut his hair every day, the High Priest every Sabbath Eve, ordinary priests once every 30 days (Babyl. Sanhedrin, 22b). And according to the Mishnah one may not have one's hair cut before the beginning of a Sabbath or a Holy Day (Shabbath, 1b). Certain hair-styles, like the growing of a forelock, were forbidden to Jews for fear of resemblance to gentile fashions (Tosefta Shabbath, 6a).

Hair treatment included washing, combing, dyeing and oiling. The practice of oiling the hair is also mentioned in the New Testament: "A woman came up to him with a jar of very expensive ointment and she poured it on his head" (Matthew, 26:7). Washing the hair regularly was also a way of getting rid of lice, which certainly bothered most of the

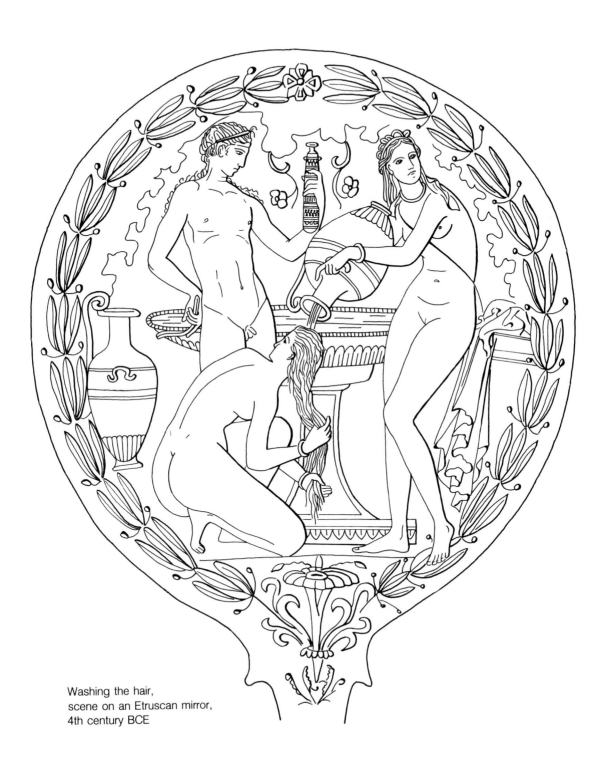

Washing the hair,
scene on an Etruscan mirror,
4th century BCE

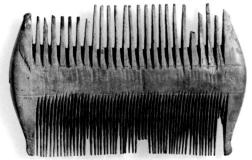

Wooden comb, Jericho area ,Roman period

populace in ancient times. A recent examination of wooden combs from Qumran and the Judaean Desert revealed traces of numerous lice and their eggs attached to them. One way of fighting this infestation was greasing the hair with oil, for oil prevents the penetration of oxygen and thus suffocates the lice.

Gray hair was considered a sign of old age, and women tried to eliminate or conceal white hairs that showed up on their heads, as recounted in the Talmud: "Seeing a single white hair, she plucked it out" (Jerus. *Shabbath*, 6a [7d]). Dyeing the hair was common practice. Josephus relates that when King Herod grew old and wanted to hide his age, he started dyeing his hair black (*Ant.*, 16, 233). Even the dyeing of beards was known among the Jews (Babyl. *Baba Metzia*, 60b).

We have much more evidence on hair fashions in the Greco-Roman world, preserved on statues and coins and in the numerous paintings on vases. In classical Greece men and women would let their hair grow long, and only servants and slaves, as well as mourners, would cut their hair. The hair billowed down over shoulders and back, and at times was tied with a narrow ribbon or braided into plaits. The men fastened their hair with a simple ribbon, while the women preferred diadems. Wealthy women wore gold diadems or a string of pearls, and some laced gold threads through their hair. One of the most prevalent hair-styles for women was the parting in the middle with the hair combed to the sides. Hair braided into plaits would be wound around the head, or gathered into a bun and fastened with a gold pin, and some women gathered it into a net. It was customary to cover part of the forehead with hair, for a low, narrow forehead was considered beautiful. Among the Greeks, most of whom were dark-haired, blond hair was much admired, and women with dark hair dyed it with various preparations, or exposed it to the sun for hours on end in order to bleach it. In the early periods, Greek men wore beards, but from the 4th century BCE on, the time of Alexander the Great, they were clean-shaven and only elderly men cultivated their beards and mustaches. During this time hair-styles also changed: from now on the haircuts of ordinary citizens were short and curly, while the aristocrats continued growing their hair long. Roman men shaved their beards until Emperor Hadrian, in the 2nd century CE, brought beards back into fashion. The shaving of a youth's beard for the first time was accompanied by a family celebration, and from the time of Augustus on this event was marked by a public ceremony, at which the shorn curls were dedicated to the gods. Sometimes they were put into a casket and kept at home as a precious memento.

Among Roman women arranging the hair was a matter of great importance. Though in the Republican period hair-styles were relatively simple – the hair was combed back and gathered in a bun fastened with a pin – in the Imperial period, with the new emphasis on ostentation in external appearance, the art of hair design reached its apogee. The hair-styles became complicated and intricate, sometimes to the point of exaggeration. It was fashionable to have a parting in the middle, or two parallel partings. The central

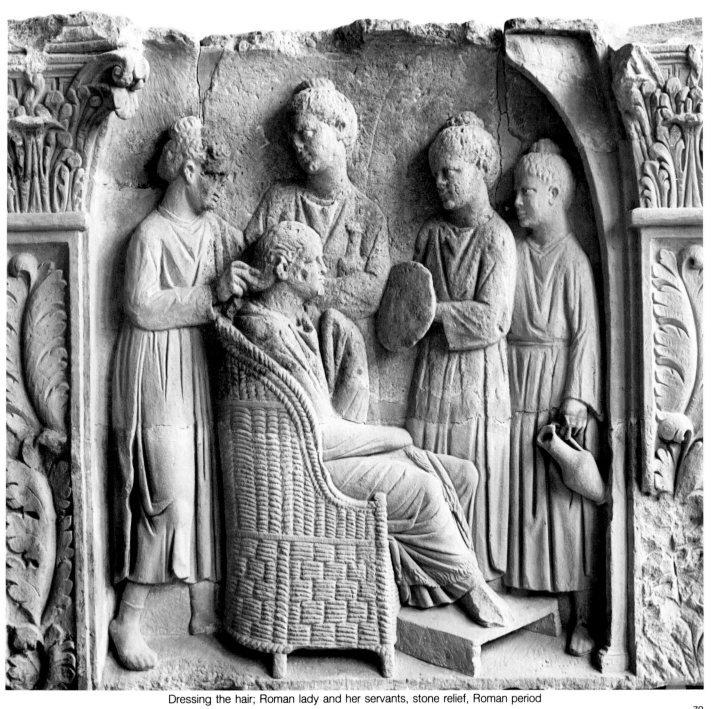

Dressing the hair; Roman lady and her servants, stone relief, Roman period

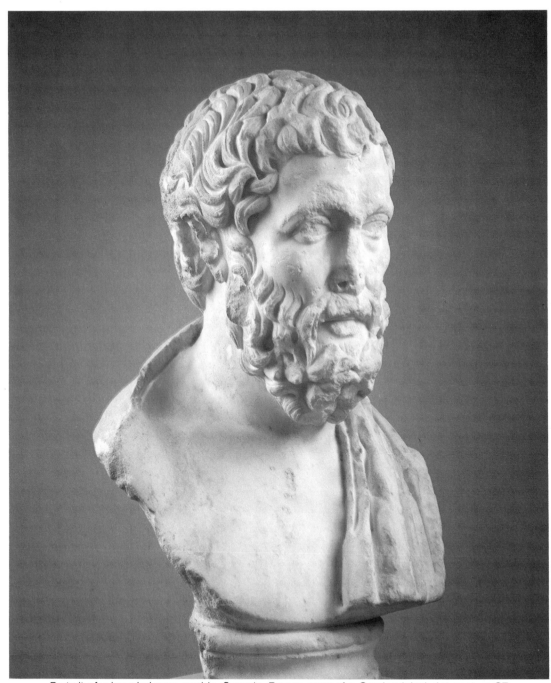

Portrait of a bearded man, marble, Samaria, Roman copy of a Greek original, 1st century CE

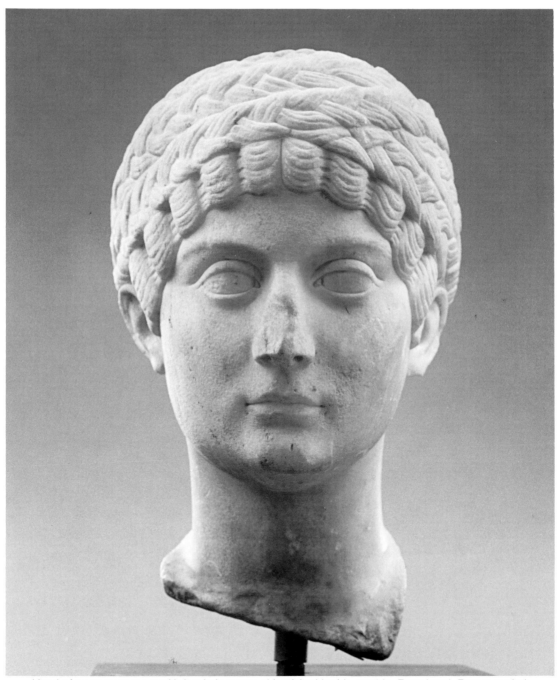

Head of a young woman with her hair arranged in plaited braids, marble, Eretz Israel, Roman period

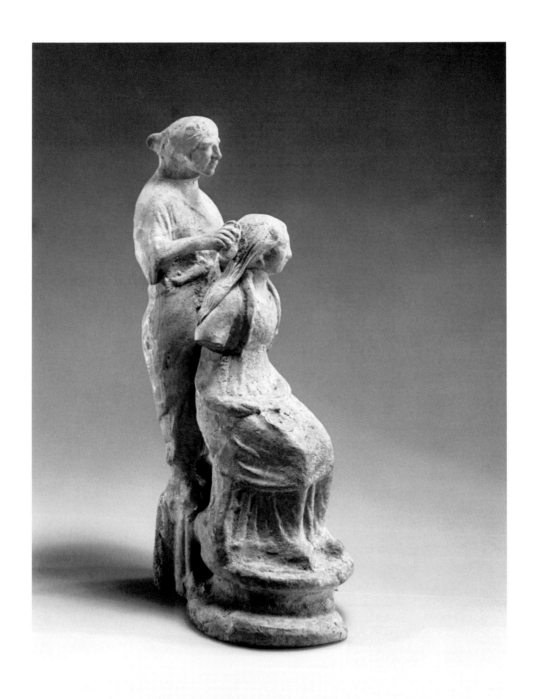

Woman having her hair combed by a maidservant, pottery figurine, Asia Minor, 2nd century BCE

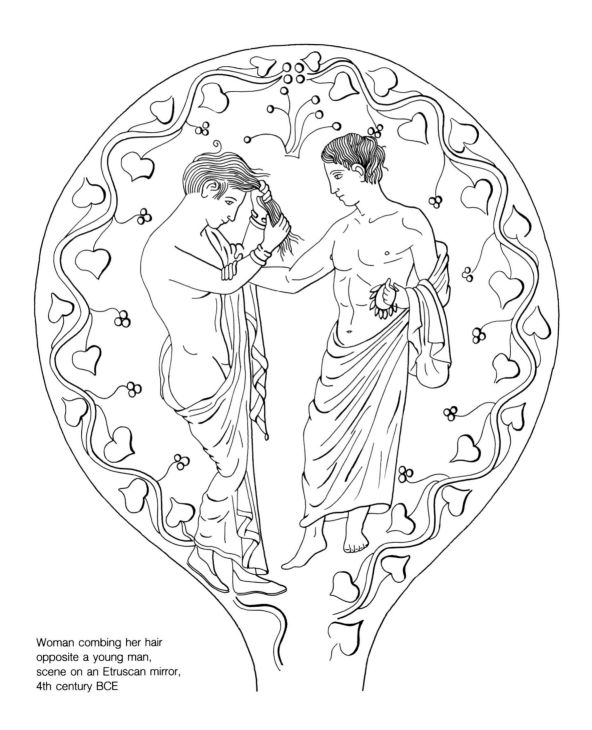

Woman combing her hair
opposite a young man,
scene on an Etruscan mirror,
4th century BCE

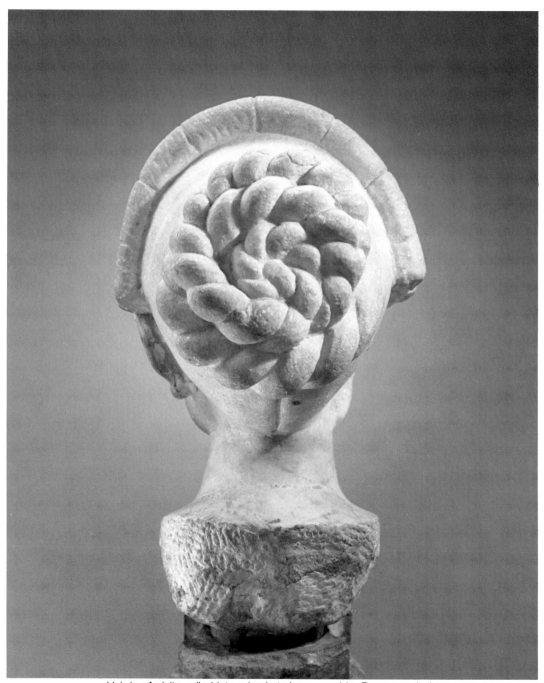

Hairdo of plaits coiled into a basket shape, marble, Roman period

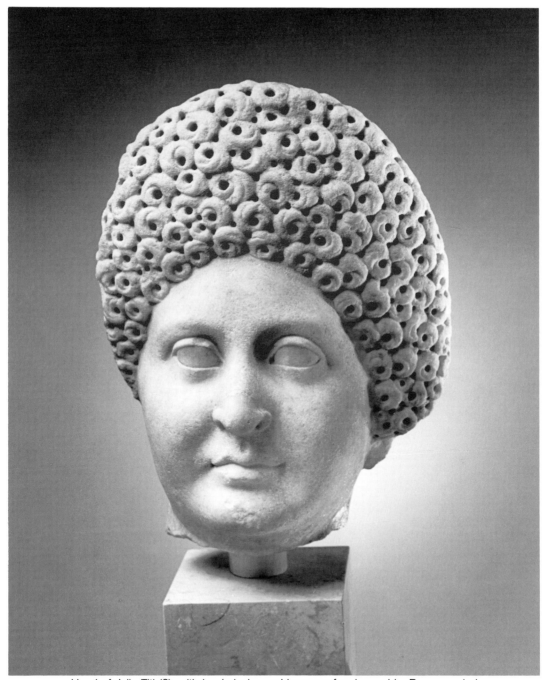

Head of Julia Titi (?), with her hair dressed in rows of curls, marble, Roman period

strip of hair was rolled forward into a kind of ball and the rest of the hair was combed back and tied into a bun. Most favored were coiffures of curls arranged in graded rows, one on top of the other, in something like a tall structure. Another hairdo was made of braided plaits which were wound around the head or braided from behind into plaits and then coiled into a basket form. Women whose hair had thinned, or who were tired of dyeing it, wore blond wigs – the color most in demand. The hair was dyed with various compounds, including a soap that the Gauls developed for dyeing the hair red (Pliny, *Nat. Hist.*, XXVIII:191). From the time of Hadrian on, it became customary to wear wigs, whether full or partial ones. These wigs were so well-made that it was difficult to distinguish them from natural hair.

The Roman lady had a private hairdresser *(tonstrix)* or a special maidservant who had gained expertise at hairdressing, and the treatment took many hours. On a stone relief from the Roman period we see a lady sitting on a chair with four servants around her: one is arranging her hair, another holds a mirror up to her, while the third holds a flask. The general populace, men as well as women, enjoyed the services of the numerous barbers and hairdressers in the city. As people spent many hours there, barber-shops became a meeting-place and center for the exchange of gossip. Around the walls benches were arranged, where people sat to await their turn, and on the walls hung mirrors for the clients to inspect their hairdos. The barber was assisted by apprentices, whom wealthy Romans sent to him to acquire expertise.

Among archaeological material from Palestine there are various implements that were used for hair treatment such as combs, hairpins, razors, and the like. The comb is known from as early as the Natufian period. The earliest combs were made of ivory and bone, and from the historical periods on they were mostly made of wood. Most of the combs are two-sided: one side with closely spaced teeth, the other with more widely spaced teeth, just like the combs of today. Especially common among the finds are hairpins, which were used to pin up the hair or to adorn the hairdo. These are made of bone, ivory, or metal, and their heads were generally carved in shapes of animals or humans. "Haircurlers" of the Egyptian type, from the Late Canaanite period, have also been found. These curlers consist of two arms; the hair was wound around one of these, and was then pushed into a slot in the other arm. Curlers of a different type were metal coils, known from classical times, which served to ornament locks of curls. The razors were used to shave both the beard and the head. Most of the razors which have been preserved are of the Egyptian type, from the Late Canaanite period. Additional items from the Roman period on are scissors and tweezers. The latter were used to pluck unwanted hairs and formed part of the regular toilet equipment.

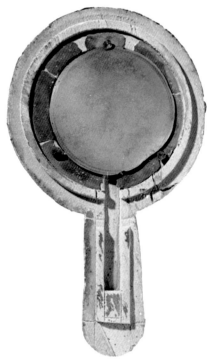

Bronze mirror in a wooden case, Cave of Letters, Judaean Desert, Roman period

An item which no woman could do without was the mirror. Mirrors were made of metal burnished and polished until one could see one's reflection in it. Apart from their use in making up the face and arranging the hair, mirrors are often shown in Egyptian reliefs and wall paintings in the context of funerary cults, either held up before the deceased, or placed in his hand or under his chair. Depictions of mirrors in everyday use are especially prevalent in Greek art – on tombstones and statues, and especially in vase paintings. These depict domestic scenes in which the woman is seen holding a mirror in her hand, and in some the mirror is seen hanging on the wall.

The mirrors that have survived from the ancient East were mostly made of copper or bronze and were polished on one side. Most were cast in one piece with the tang, which was then inserted into a handle of bone, ivory, wood, alabaster, or faience. From the archaeological evidence and the written records it appears that Egypt was a center of the mirror industry during the Middle and Late Bronze Ages, in the 2nd millennium BCE, though polished mirrors are known from as early as the mid-3rd millennium.

In Egypt the gleaming mirror was regarded as a symbol of the sun, and the reflection of the human image symbolized vitality, generation and regeneration. The mirror disk, which was usually of copper or bronze, and sometimes of gold or silver, was originally egg-shaped or cordiform, and in the course of time became circular. The handle, usually shaped like a papyrus stalk or a lotus plant, was sometimes crowned with the head of the goddess Hathor or the figure of the god Bes. Some handles were designed in the shape of a nude female whose arms were either resting along her body or spread out to the sides. To protect the mirror, it was customary to wrap it in a piece of fabric or keep it in a sheath or in a special box, together with all the other cosmetic preparations. In the tomb of Tut-Ankh-Amon a splendid wooden mirror-case has been found.

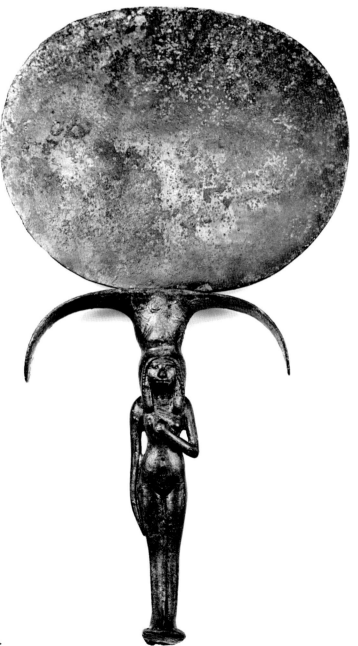

Mirror of an Egyptian type with handle in the shape of a woman carrying a mirror disk on her head, bronze, Akko, 14th century BCE ▷

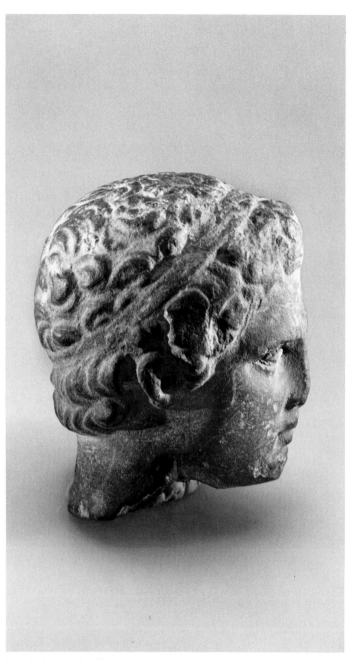

Head of a youth with a ribbon in his curly hair, stone, Eretz Israel, Hellenistic period

Mirrors dating from the Late Bronze Age (15th–13th centuries BCE) have been found in Palestine – at Tell el-Ajjul, Megiddo, Akko, Deir el-Balah and other sites, and most probably they originated in Egypt. Only few mirrors are known from the Iron Age, while from the Persian period (6th–4th centuries BCE) many mirrors have been found in tombs. These are round and polished disks of metal with a bronze handle decorated with a spiral design. Only in rare cases has the handle been preserved into which the tang was inserted, as in the bone-handled mirror from Atlit.

In the course of the centuries, a wide variety of mirrors was produced, to cater to the tastes and needs of female and male clients of all classes. The mirror disks were made of various metals, from copper and bronze to silver, or silvered and gilded. Etruscan mirrors, decorated with engraved designs on the back, became popular in the late 6th century BCE. These decorations, their subjects usually taken from Greek mythology, are often of a high artistic level and excellent technical standard. From the 3rd century BCE on, the backs of the mirrors were convex to protect the fine designs from being disfigured by scratches when the mirror was laid down.

The mirrors from the classical Greek period are round and have a bronze handle or foot in the shape of a human figure. Towards the end of the 5th century BCE, mirrors consisting of two parts – a polished face and a cover – became popular in Greece. The cover, which was often decorated with engraved concentric circles, protected the face from damage. Mirrors of this type became most popular in the Hellenistic period.

From the Roman period onwards it became customary to keep mirrors in cases made of wood or bronze. These mirrors were made of silver, bronze inlaid with silver, and even of glass on a lead base. Generally, mirrors were small enough to be held in the hand, but there were also mirrors that were meant to be hung on the wall. Mirrors from the Roman period have been found in various places in Palestine, for instance among the belongings of the refugees from the time of the Bar Kokhba revolt, found in the Cave of Letters in the Judaean Desert. Apparently, even during emergencies, women were not willing to part from this essential item.

# Perfume Production

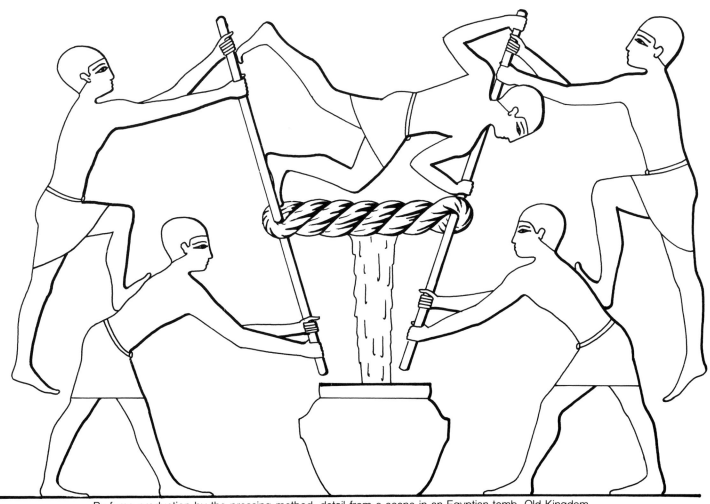

Perfume production by the pressing method, detail from a scene in an Egyptian tomb, Old Kingdom

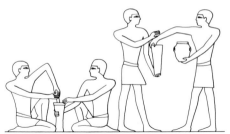

Mixing the aromatic oils in containers,
after a scene in an Egyptian tomb,
Old Kingdom

In the ancient world perfumes and spices were a precious commodity, very much in demand, and at times exceeding even silver and gold in value. They served ritual, funerary, and therapeutic purposes, as well as meeting ordinary cosmetic requirements. Their high price stemmed from the tiny quantities that could generally be extracted from the plants, the complicated processing, and the costs of transportation from afar. Perfumes were therefore a luxury product, used mainly in temples and in the homes of the noble and the wealthy, and constituted part of the royal treasures. The Judaean kings kept them in their treasure-houses (2 Kings, 20:13) together with their gold and silver. Spices were among the gifts that the Queen of Sheba brought to King Solomon in Jerusalem: "And she gave the king a hundred and twenty talents of gold, and of spices very great store, and precious stones" (1 Kings, 10:2, 10). In the Temple, too, large quantities of perfume were consumed, and among the priests there were families who specialized in the mixing and brewing of various kinds of spices and perfumes: "And some of the sons of the priests made the ointment of the spices" (1 Chronicles, 9:30).

The Bible mentions various plants, from whose flowers, fruits, leaves, bark or resin perfumes and ointments were produced: aloes (ohalot); balsam (bosem), probably the aparsemon-opobalsamum of the Second Temple period; galbanum (helbanah); henna (kopher); saffron (karkom); frankincense (levonah); ladanum (lot); myrrh (mor); stacte (nataf); gum (nekhot); spikenard (nard); balm (zori); cassia (kida, keziot); cane, calamus (kene bosem); cinnamon (kinnamon). Only a few of these plants were indigenous to Palestine: henna, saffron, balm, and ladanum. They grew in the Jordan Valley, at En Gedi (Song of Solomon, 1:14) and Gilead (Genesis, 37:25). The others were brought from distant lands such as India, Ceylon, South Arabia, and Somali.

In the Greco-Roman world the demand for spices expanded greatly in comparison to previous periods, and an extensive trade developed in these products. The Near East played a prominent part in this trade, with important trading centers at Alexandria and Mendes in Egypt, and also in Palestine.

The preparation of perfumes requires great skill and has always been the exclusive domain of specialists. Already in antiquity, however, the high price of spices led to attempts at counterfeiting them. For this reason the growers and perfumers, who were organized in closed family-based guilds, guarded the secrets of their trade jealously and passed them on as an inheritance from one generation to the next. Their high standing, and the great regard in which they were held, are reflected in a saying of the Sages: "Happy is he whose craft is that of a perfume-maker" (Babyl. Kiddushin, 82b). The perfumers had to have a highly developed sense of smell, a good memory for fragrances, and the ability to combine and reconstitute various compounds. From biblical and Mesopotamian sources we learn that women too engaged in the perfumer's craft and were employed in this capacity in temples and at the courts of kings: "This will be the way of the king . . . and he will take your daughters to be perfumers" (1 Sam., 8:11, 13).

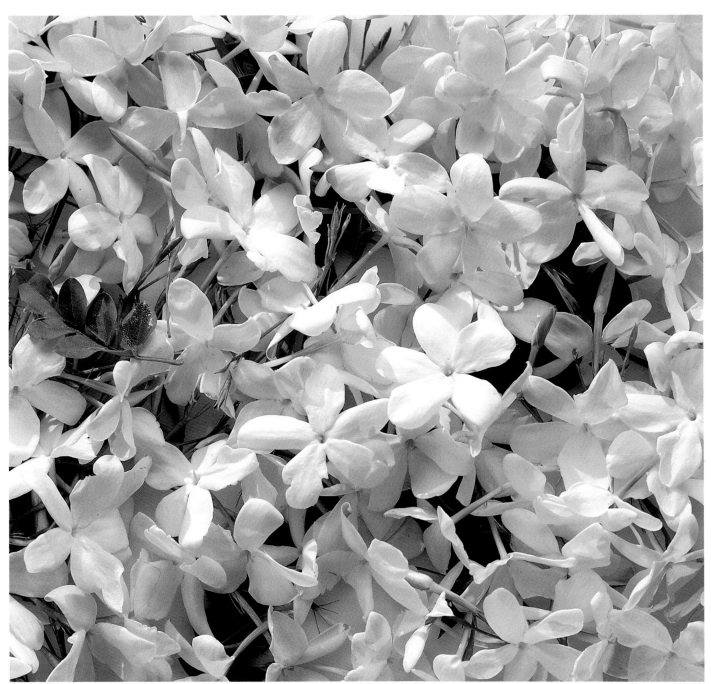

Jasmine flowers

Pressing the aromatic plants by wringing a cloth, stone relief, Egypt, 4th century BCE
▽

The craft of perfume-brewing flourished in the Roman period, during which standards of refinement and personal care reached unprecedented heights, and the consumption of cosmetics spread to broad strata of the population.

From the ancient sources we learn much about the uses of perfumes, but very few of them describe the methods of preparation. Tablets dating from the 2nd millennium BCE, found at the Mycenaean palace at Pylos in Greece, list the allocation of raw materials for perfumes, but contain no precise recipes or formulas. Assyrian records from the time of Tukulti-Ninurta I, in the second half of the 13th century BCE, do contain recipes for perfumes, as well as lists of ingredients and of the equipment necessary for producing them. Our knowledge about perfume preparation in Egypt comes from inscriptions on papyri and on walls of tombs, and often from finds in special chambers in temples where ointments and perfumes were kept. Of special interest is a wall painting in a tomb at

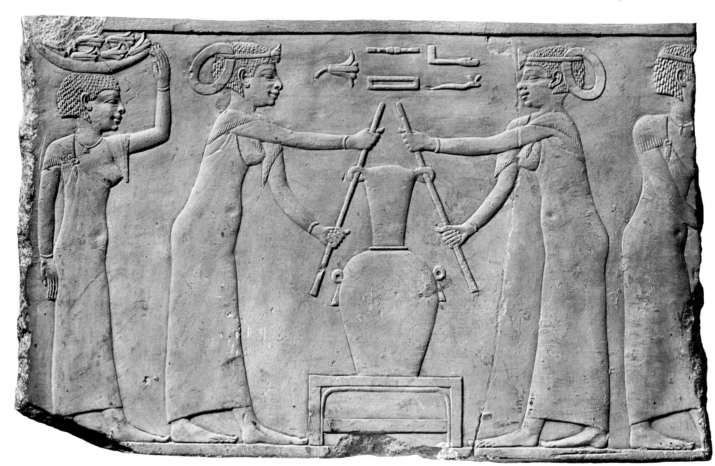

Thebes from the early 14th century BCE, which depicts a perfumer's workshop and the stages of perfume preparation.

More extensive literary information about perfume production has come to us from various classical writers. The three most important sources on this subject are the works of Theophrastus, who lived in the 4th–3rd centuries BCE; Dioscorides, from the 1st century CE; and Pliny the Elder, a contemporary of Dioscorides. Theophrastus, in his work *De Odoribus*, describes the properties of various oils and spices used in perfume production, and also the odors themselves. Dioscorides, in his *De Materia Medica*, discusses components of perfumes and their medical properties, and lists detailed recipes for perfumes. Pliny, in his *Naturalis Historia*, describes aromatic plants and perfumes in the areas where they grow. Even a depiction of the production of perfume has survived – in a wall painting in the Vetii house at Pompeii: here Cupids and Psyches are shown carrying out various stages of the processing.

Gathering lilies for perfume, stone relief, Egypt, 4th century BCE
▽

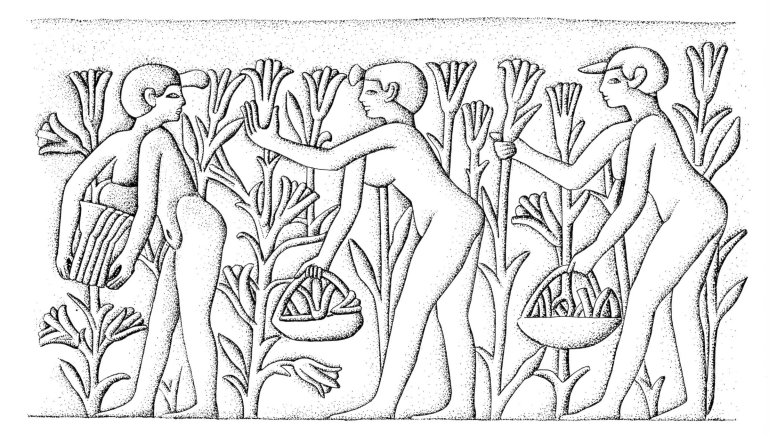

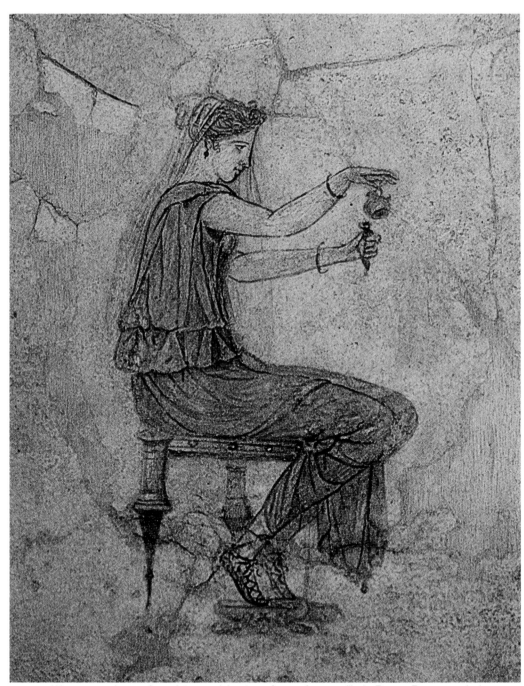

Woman pouring perfume into an alabastron, fresco from a villa in Rome, Roman period

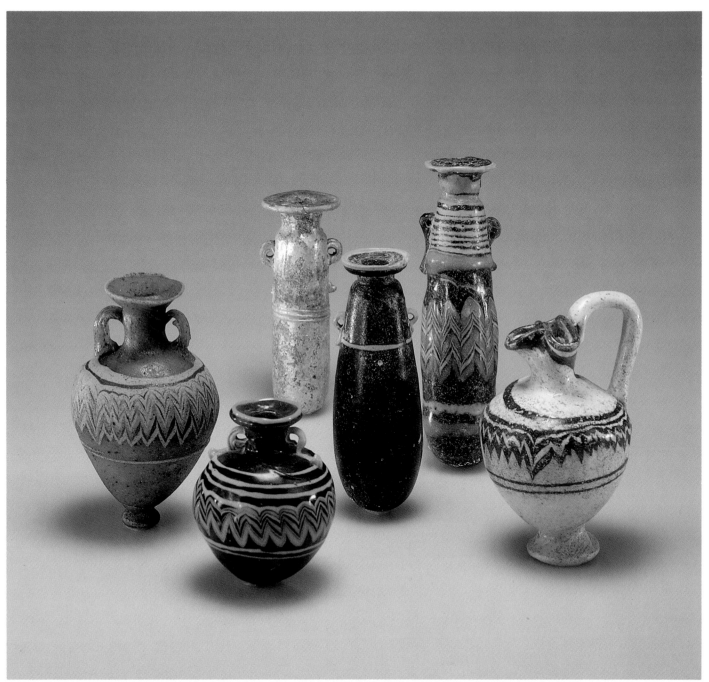

Alabastra and amphoriskoi of core-wound glass, Palestine and Syria, 6th–4th centuries BCE

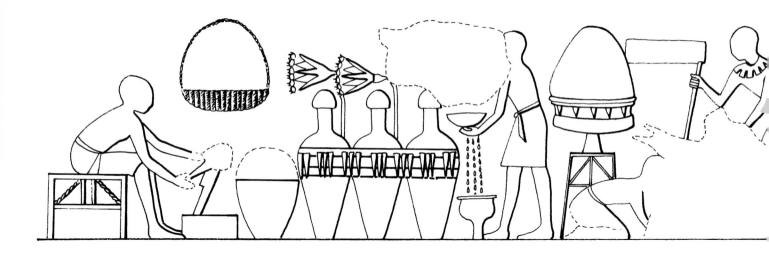

Perfume compounder's workshop. From right to left: oil jars; assistants grinding the aromatics; another assistant mixing the ground aromatics; assistant stirring the liquid in a bowl standing on an oven (?); assistant straining the liquid. At the far left, the master perfumer oversees the work. Wall painting, Egypt, early 14th century BCE

In Jerusalem, in the basement of a 1st-century CE house which overlooked the Temple, archaeologists have uncovered ovens, cooking-pots and mortars, evidence that the place had been a kind of workshop. It has been suggested that products such as perfume and incense were manufactured here for use in the Temple. A building of the 1st century CE, uncovered at En Boqeq on the shore of the Dead Sea, was identified as a workshop for producing cosmetics. The excavators suggested that cosmetics and perfumes may have been produced there from the balsam and palm trees which grew in this region.

In the production of perfumes, different parts of plants were used: flowers, leaves, branches, fruits, and resin. Resin, the most expensive of the raw materials, required special skills in handling already at the gathering stage. It was obtained by making incisions in the bark of the tree, after which the resin exuded from the trunk in viscous drops. On contact with the air these hardened into tear-shaped drops, which were used as an ingredient in the production of cosmetics.

Most of the perfumes in the ancient world were made on an oil base, unlike modern perfumes, which use an alcohol base. In Palestine, the base was most often olive oil, in Mesopotamia it was sesame oil, in Anatolia linseed oil, while in Egypt mostly animal fats were used. The plant-parts were steeped in cold or hot oil, which absorbed the aromatic materials that were then stabilized by the fatty base. Pliny notes that the fattier the solution, as for example a solution based on almond oil, the more stable the perfume (Pliny, *Nat. Hist.*, XIII:19).

The first stage in the production of perfume was chopping up the herbs or the other plant-parts. Next came one of three main processing methods: pressing, cold steeping (enfleurage), and hot steeping (maceration).

*The pressing method* seems to have been the earliest. First the plant-parts were crushed, in the same way as olives or grapes were pressed, i.e., in a basin. This method is depicted

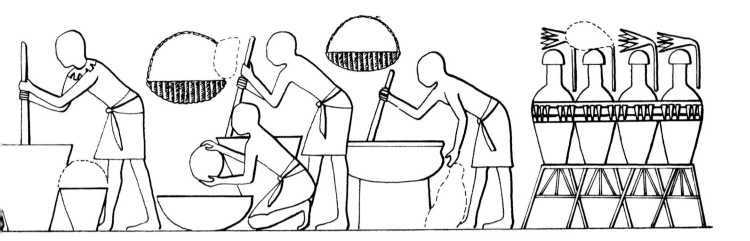

in Egyptian tomb paintings from the 3rd millennium BCE, and we can trace improvements developing in the course of time. The aromatic materials were placed in a folded cloth which had loops at both ends. Into each of these loops a rod was thrust, and the rods were then twisted in opposite directions, thus pressing the contents. The main disadvantage of this method was that it did not enable the extraction of all the aromatic ingredients from the plant-parts. Indeed, it seems to have been used only in pre-classical periods.

*Cold steeping (enfleurage)* was the easiest and most convenient method, and though it was not suitable for all plants, it was especially effective with flowers of a certain kind, such as jasmine, roses, and others. In this method, the petals were spread on a layer of animal fat placed between two boards, like a press. When the scent had been absorbed by the fat, after about 24 hours, the petals were thrown away and replaced by fresh ones. This process was repeated daily, sometimes for several weeks, until the fat was saturated with scent. At the end of the process, a perfumed pomade was obtained. In Egyptian paintings, women attending banquets are depicted with cones of

Cupids and Psyches carrying out various phases of perfume production, fresco in villa at Pompeii (Vetii House), 1st century CE

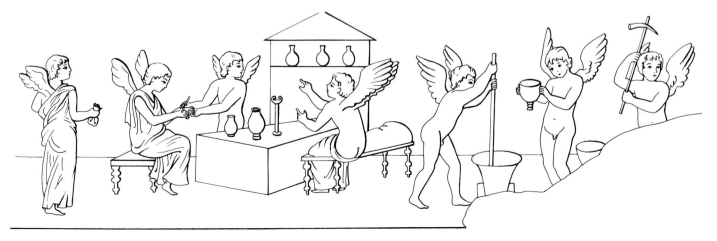

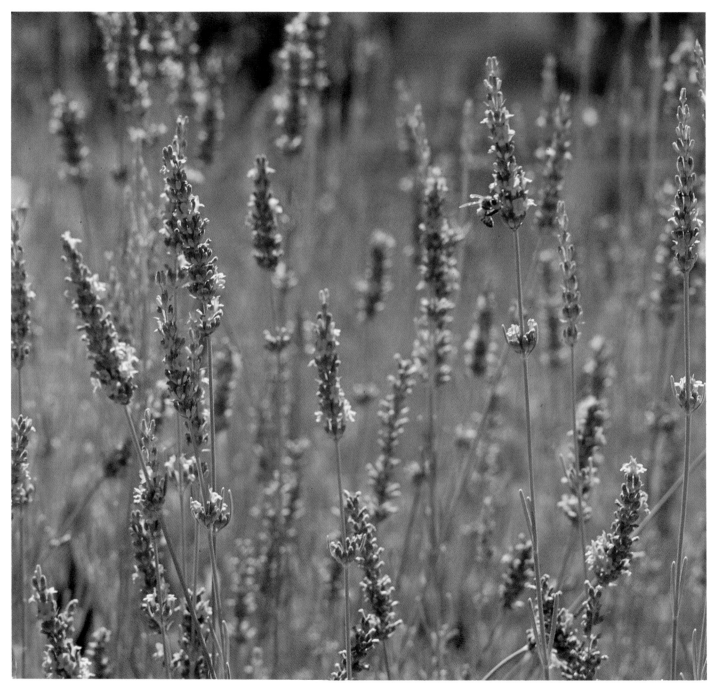

Lavender flowers

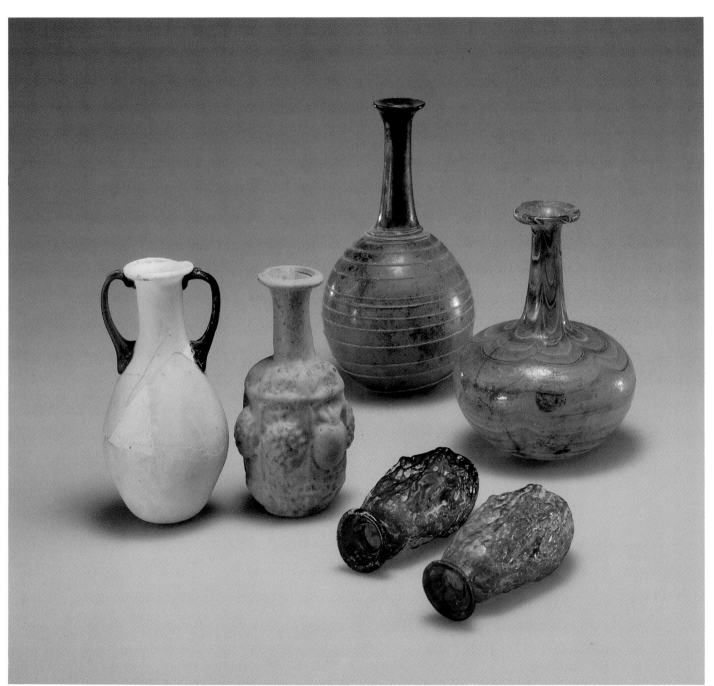

Perfume bottles, glass, Eretz Israel, 1st century CE

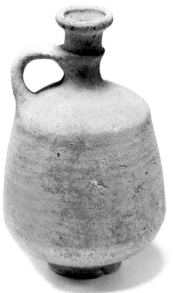

Decanter with ridged neck,
for storing precious liquids,
pottery, Eretz Israel,
8th–7th centuries BCE

pomade on their heads. This method has been in use until recently, though in modern times, when the saturation of the fat was complete, it was washed with alcohol and strained.

*Hot steeping (maceration)* was the method most commonly used in the perfume industry. In this process, the oil was pre-treated by the addition of a solution of astringent materials mixed with wine or water. Theophrastus notes that this stage was particularly essential when the base used was olive oil, which does not retain odors well, or when the aromatic material was particularly volatile (Theophrastus, *De Odoribus*, 14, 17, 55).

In this pre-treated oil the plant-parts or resin were steeped, and the mixtures heated to a temperature of 65° Celsius. The jars of oil were heated in vats of boiling water (i.e., a double-boiler method), and not over an open flame, to prevent the perfume from evaporating rapidly or absorbing scorched smells from the fire. The heated mixture was left to stand for several days, and it was stirred occasionally; then the floral components were strained off, and fresh ones were added. Sometimes dyes were added to the mixture during the steeping process. When the aromatic materials were completely absorbed, the perfume was strained one last time and decanted into containers.

The finished product was kept in a cool and shady place in containers of lead or alabaster, which keep their contents cool. When a woman wanted to try the perfume, she would dab a little on the back of her hand rather than on the warm palm, so as not to spoil its quality.

The process of perfume production as we learn of it from the Pylos tablets is basically similar to the methods used during the classical period, and especially interesting is the use of wool for straining the perfume. From Assyrian records we get a slightly different picture. Here the aromatic ingredients were steeped in hot water during the day. In the evening more spices were added to the mixture, which was then left to stand overnight. The next day the mixture was reheated, perhaps after a straining and an addition of spices. Oil was added only at the end of the steeping process, after which the entire mixture was stirred. The vessel was then covered and heated to complete the mixing of the oil with all the other ingredients. After this the residue that had accumulated was removed from the vessel, the mixture was stirred again, and the vessel was covered and left standing for four days. Finally the mixture was boiled once more, evidently on a low flame, and after cooling it was strained and decanted into flasks. It appears that in this process, in contrast to methods practiced in later periods, the oil was not pre-treated by the addition of astringents, and the aromatic ingredients were absorbed by the hot water. The entire mixture was heated directly over a fire and not in a double boiler.

Egyptian depictions furnish abundant material concerning the stages of perfume production. In them we see women expressing the aromatic essence from the flowers of the lily, and oil merchants carrying their products in animal skins; in their hands are funnels for pouring the precious liquid into smaller containers. Most interesting is a tomb painting from Thebes, which depicts a perfumer's workshop and the different stages of his work. Here we see assistants grinding the aromatic materials, one mixing the ground components with oil in a large basin, and another stirring the liquid in a basin that stands on top of a stove. Yet another figure holds a strainer through which he pours a liquid in which aromatic ingredients have probably been steeped. The master perfumer himself sits to the side and oversees the work.

When we compare the various ancient descriptions of perfume production, we see that the process remained essentially unchanged for more than a thousand years. In fact, some of the methods described were still employed in the early 20th century.

The equipment required for perfume manufacture was similar to that of an ordinary kitchen: basins and pots for steeping, heating, and mixing; large jars for storing the oil; mortars and pestles for crushing the aromatic substances; bowls for the various herbs, juglets for storing the resin; strainers; wooden or bone spoons for stirring; and jugs and jars for the finished product. Presumably only a little of the quantity produced was decanted into small flasks, while the greater part was poured into larger containers, suitable for delivery to various destinations. This assumption is suggested by the finds at Pylos, where stirrup-jars of various sizes were discovered. The stirrup-jar has a low biconical body, two loop handles, a closed false neck and a spout on the shoulder – all features especially suitable for storing precious liquids: the jar can be filled and emptied only through the spout, and the liquid poured from it will come out slowly, drop by drop. The closed neck was designed to prevent the liquid from spilling during transportation. The assumption is that the large stirrup-jars were used for transporting the perfumes, while the exquisitely made small stirrup-jars were intended to hold perfumes for personal use.

At sites from the First Temple period in Eretz Israel, another type of vessel – the decanter – has frequently been found. This jug has a carinated shoulder and a high, narrow, often ridged neck. These features also make the decanter well suited for storing and transporting precious liquids, and since this vessel has been found in large quantities at En Gedi, which was a perfume-producing center (see below), it is possible that, like the stirrup-jar, it too was used for marketing perfumes.

Just as the art of the perfumer required skill, refinement, and a discriminating taste, so too did the art of fashioning vessels for the perfumes. The artists gave their imagination free rein and created vessels of alabaster, glass, ivory, and metal, in addition to pottery. The commonest container for perfume was the small pottery jar or amphoriskos, with a small, usually spherical body, a long, thin neck, and a narrow, easily stoppered mouth, which made it possible to pour the liquid in a very fine stream. The drawback of pottery, however, was that the odor of the liquid would evaporate through the porous clay, thus

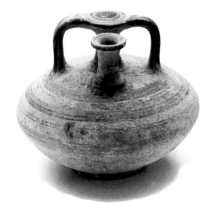

Stirrup jar for perfume (?) with closed neck and spout, pottery, 14th century BCE

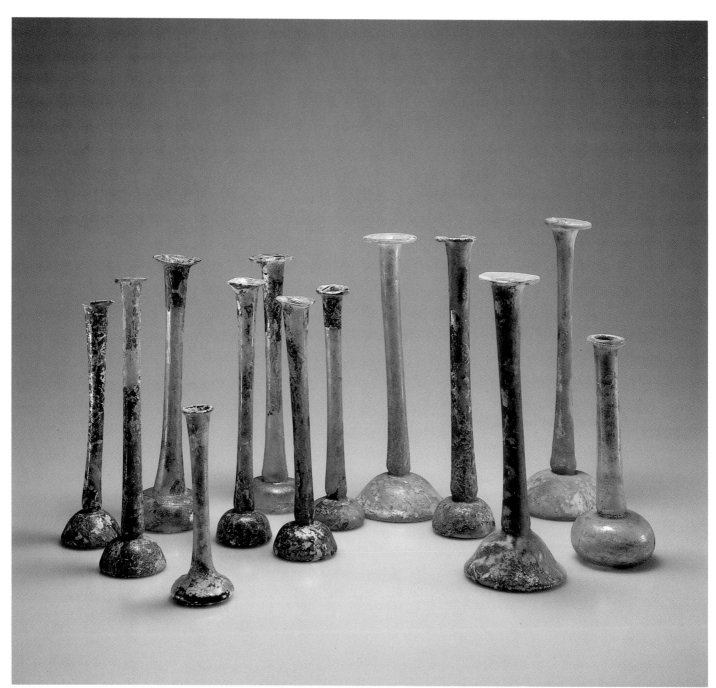

'Candlestick' glass perfume bottles, Eretz Israel, 1st–3rd centuries CE

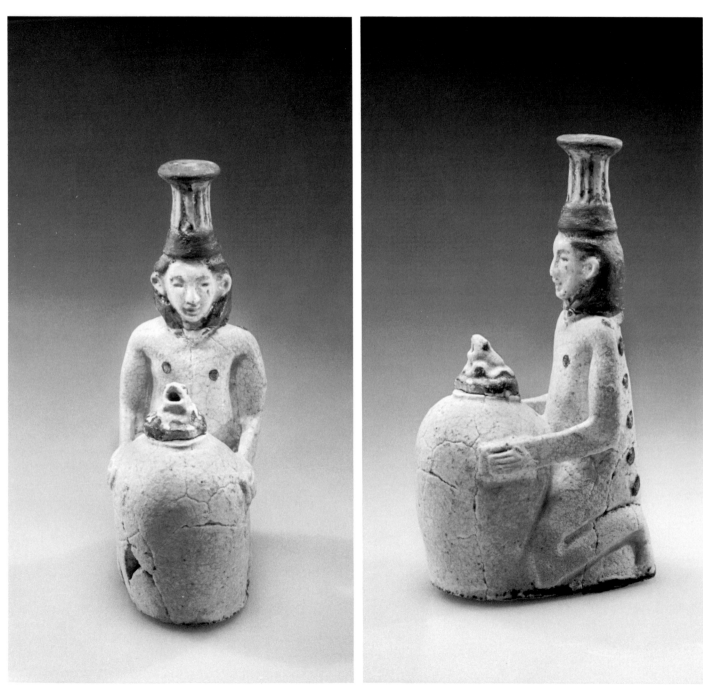

Perfume bottle in the shape of a kneeling woman, faience, 7th century BCE

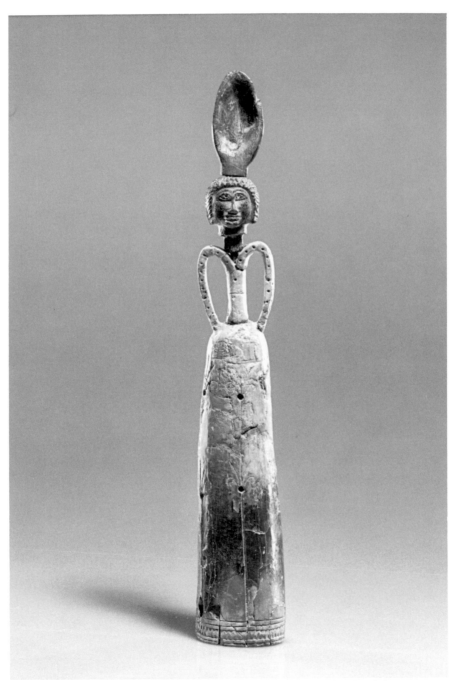

Perfume bottle in the shape of a woman with a spoon on her head, ivory,
Lachish, 13th century BCE

impairing its quality. Indeed, as early as the middle of the 2nd millennium BCE, the Egyptians began imitating the shape of the pottery juglet in multi-colored core-wound glass vessels. Between the 6th and the 4th centuries BCE, small flasks made of colored glass spread to many places along the Mediterranean coasts, and were probably used for perfumes. It is clear that the expensive perfumes were marketed in elegant containers made of glass, pottery, and other materials, some of them animal-shaped, others shaped like pomegranates. One especially beautiful artifact is an ivory bottle in the shape of a woman, from the Late Canaanite period, found in the Fosse Temple at Lachish. It is cylindrical, with a long narrow neck ending in a female head, which carries a spoon. When the bottle was tilted, a few drops of liquid would drip onto the spoon, ready for use, and when it was righted, the remaining drops would flow back inside. Bronze perfume bottles shaped like robed women are known from Iran in the Achaemenian period. The women's heads feature an intricate coiffure, the top part of which serves as a lid that is attached to the flask by a chain. Bottles in the shape of women made of ivory, bone, and metal were popular in the ancient East between the 7th and 5th centuries BCE. A distinctive type is the vessel shaped like a kneeling woman between whose legs is a large jar with a frog on top. From the mouth of the frog the precious liquid is poured. The woman's back is decorated with brown dots. Though these vessels originate in Egypt, many have been found in the Western Mediterranean area, and some consider them a "Phoenician" product, dating from the 7th century BCE.

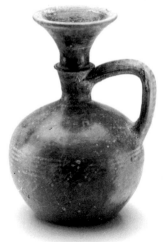

Perfume juglet of the Cypro-Phoenician type, pottery, Eretz Israel, 9th–8th centuries BCE

As already noted, stone vessels were particularly suitable as perfume containers, and among these the most common was the alabastron, named after the alabaster from which it was generally made, though it also exists in pottery and glass. Its narrow neck and broad rim facilitated a controlled pouring of the liquid it contained. One could drip some perfume from it onto a finger or into a small bowl, or alternatively dip a small stick into it and use that to dab perfume on the body. Greek vase paintings often show women in various postures holding an alabastron.

The perfume flask industry developed most extensively in Greece, where especially beautiful vessels were produced, some ornamented with marvelous paintings and others in the shape of animals or female heads. The invention of blown glass in the 1st century BCE led to a revolution in perfume containers. Glass, because of its beauty, its impermeability and its light weight, quickly replaced the pottery flasks, and from then on the small glass flask became the distinctive receptacle for perfume, as it is to this day. This change is reflected in the archaeological finds, and many glass flasks have been found, not only in tombs, as funerary offerings, but in domestic settings as well. The most widespread type was the perfume flask with a long narrow neck, like that of the pottery flask, to reduce the evaporation of the perfume (Mishnah *Parah*, 12:2).

From the 1st and 2nd centuries CE onwards, flasks made of mold-blown glass of distinctive shapes became common. Among these we find bottles shaped like fruits such as dates, which may have been intended to designate the contents of the flask.

Pomegranate-shaped perfume bottles.
On the right: glass, Cyprus (?),
14th–13th centuries BCE;
on the left: pottery, Eretz Israel,
9th–8th centuries BCE

The narrow mouth of the perfume flask could be stoppered with a piece of cloth, parchment, or papyrus: "He who takes out an already collected bond . . . to wrap around a small perfume bottle" (Tosefta *Shabbath*, 8:12).

Unfortunately, only a few of the numerous bottles found contain any residue of their original contents. In two glass bottles of the 2nd–3rd centuries CE, probably from the Jerusalem area, the residue was analyzed and identified as olive oil. This may indicate that the flask originally contained perfume, since in Palestine perfumes were generally made on an olive oil base, which was all that remained in these bottles after the aromatic substances had evaporated.

Many of the plants that were used in the production of perfumes and ointments in the ancient world are mentioned in the Bible. These include spikenard (Song of Solomon, 1:12), which was one of the most costly perfumes. In the Talmud it is referred to as *foliatum*. A "flask of *foliatum*" (Mishnah *Shabbath*, 6:3) is a synonym for an expensive flask of perfume. Spikenard is identified with the plant *Nardostachys Jatamansi*, which grows in the Himalayas.

A perfume in wide use was myrrh, which existed in liquid form – "oil of myrrh" – and in crystalline form – "pure myrrh." It was used in the preparation of "the oil of holy ointment" (Exodus, 30:23–25), and also for perfuming the body and the clothes: "Thy garments are fragrant with myrrh and aloes and cassia" (Psalms, 45:9). Myrrh was also used therapeutically. In the New Testament we read that Jesus, before his crucifixion, was offered wine mingled with myrrh (Mark, 15:23), perhaps to alleviate the pain. Myrrh is generally identified with *Commiphora Abyssinica* and also with *Commiphora Schimperi*, trees or shrubs that grow in Africa and South Arabia.

Frankincense is mentioned frequently in the Bible and the Talmud as one of the most important ingredients of incense (Leviticus, 2:15; 24:7), but it was used mainly in funerary rites, and also for healing and cosmetics. It was extracted from trees of the *Boswellia* species, which grow in Somalia and South Arabia. On other uses of myrrh and frankincense, see "The Spice Trade."

Galbanum was another ingredient of the incense used in the Tabernacle, together with onycha and stacte (Exodus, 30:34–35). It is extracted from the stems and roots of the plant *Ferula Galbaniflua* or *Ferula Rubricaulis*. Stacte is identified with storax, and was used in the cosmetics industry as an astringent; it has been suggested that this is a general term for different types of resins.

Cinnamon, too, was a component of the "oil of holy ointment," together with myrrh, calamus, and cassia (Exodus, 30:23). It was produced from the *Cinnamomum Zeylanicum* tree, which grows in Ceylon and Southern India.

The calamus, also known as "sweet cane," is a costly plant brought from India, and is identified with *Cymbopogon Martini* or with *Andropogon Nardus*. The cassia of Exodus 30:24 (Hebrew *kidah*) is identified with *Iris Florentina*, which grew in the Near East and is still used for producing aromatic powders.

Saffron (Song of Solomon, 4:14), identified with *Crocus Sativus* or *Crocus Longa*, is a small Mediterranean plant. The other cassia, of Psalm 45:9 (Hebrew *keziot),* is a tree similar to the cinnamon tree and is identified with *Cinnamomum Cassia*, which originated in China. The "camphire" (Song of Solomon, 1:14), more familiarly known as henna, grew in the En Gedi area. It is identified with *Lawsonia Alba* and with *Lawsonia Inermis*, a small tree or shrub with fragrant flowers. It yields a fragrant yellowish-red dye used – then as now – to dye the hair, as well as the fingernails and the palms of the hands.

Ladanum, balm, and gum are mentioned together in the Bible as the load carried by the camels of the Ishmaelites on their passage from Gilead to Egypt (Genesis, 37:25). Many identify balm with *Balanites Aegyptiaca*, a tree common in the Dead Sea area and in the Jordan Valley. The ladanum gum-resin is produced from the plants *Cistus Ladaniferus* and *Cistus Creticus*, which grow in the Mediterranean region, and the resin called *nekhot* comes from the *Astragalus* shrub, which grows in mountainous areas in Asia.

The plant called *bosem* in the Bible (Song of Solomon, 5:1) is identified by many authorities with the *opobalsamum* (Hebrew *aparsemon*) of the Second Temple period. During that period the balsam tree, which grew in the Jericho Valley and in the En Gedi orchards, was the most famous of all the plants growing in Eretz Israel. In Greek the tree was called *Balsamon* and in Latin *Balsamum* or *Opobalsamum*, and it is commonly assumed that the Hebrew name *aparsemon* is a corruption of *opobalsamum*, which means "the juice of the balsam." In point of fact we have no certain knowledge what this *aparsemon* was, but some authorities identify it with *Commiphora Opobalsamon*, of the *Burseracea* family, a plant which grows in South Arabia and Somalia. At any rate, it is evidently not the tropical persimmon fruit, the *Diospyros*, which is cultivated today. A species of the balsam shrub that grows today in South Arabia, Yemen, and Somalia is no longer used for perfume, but serves as a remedy against snake and scorpion bites.

The *aparsemon* is frequently referred to in Talmudic and classical sources as one of the most famous and precious perfumes of the ancient world (Pliny, *Nat. Hist.*, XII:111–124; Dioscorides, *De Materia Medica*, I, 19:1). Strabo writes: "Hiericus . . . is a plain . . . and is everywhere watered with streams . . . here are also the palace and the balsam park . . . accordingly it is costly and also for the reason that it is produced nowhere else" (Strabo, *Geography*, XVI:2, 41). According to Josephus, balsam seedlings were brought into Eretz Israel by the Queen of Sheba, among her gifts to King Solomon (*Antiquities*, VIII:174). It would appear that the special climatic conditions of the Dead Sea area, with

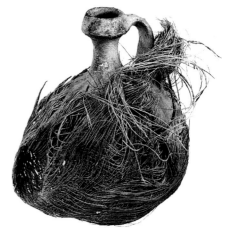

Pottery juglet wrapped in palm fibers, found containing oily liquid (*aparsemon*), discovered in a cave in the Qumran area, 1st century CE

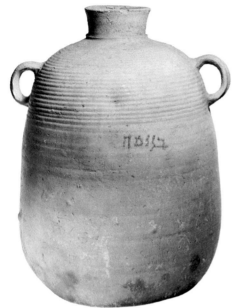

Store jar bearing the inscription
"baisamah/balsam," pottery,
Eretz Israel, 1st century CE

its high temperatures, low humidity, and minimal rain, were especially suitable for the cultivation of this unique aromatic plant. Indeed, in the Talmudic period, the area of its cultivation extended "from En-Gedi to Ramah" (Babyl. *Shabbath,* 26a).

The great economic importance of balsam is mentioned by Josephus, who records that "Antony gave Cleopatra the palm-grove at Jericho in which the balsam is produced" (*War,* 1:361). The balsam orchards had indeed been the property of the Roman Caesars and later, the "Nassi," the President of the Sanhedrin, also called "Rabbi." There is a Talmudic ruling that says: "The benediction 'who createst fragrant woods' is said only over the balsam trees of Rabbi's household and the balsam trees of Caesar's household" (Babyl. *Berakhot,* 43a). Since the balsam was so expensive, the secrets of its cultivation and production were closely guarded. Pliny records that at the time of Alexander the Great its price was double that of silver. He also writes that in 70 CE, when the army of Titus, advancing on Jerusalem, was approaching the balsam-growing area, the Jews wanted to chop down the precious orchards to prevent their falling into the hands of the enemy (Pliny, *Nat. Hist.,* XII:111). Nevertheless, the Roman army did capture the orchards, and on his return to Rome Titus displayed balsam trees in his triumphal procession.

Theophrastus too writes about the cultivation of the balsam tree. According to him, balsam was produced in "the Valley of Syria" (he was probably referring to the Dead Sea area), from an evergreen tree "as tall as a good-sized pomegranate and much branched . . . the fruit is like that of the terebinth in size shape and color and this too is very fragrant . . . and can be sold for a good price" (Theophrastus, *Hist. Plant.,* IX, 6:1–4).

The most important material derived from the tree was the sap, a viscous and sweet-smelling resin. Pliny describes how the sap was collected: "Incisions are made in the shrub and the drops exuded from the cut are collected, by means of tufts in small horns, and poured out of them into a few earthenware vessels to store . . . it was considered a fair whole day's work in summer to fill a single shell." Pliny distinguishes between three varieties of balsam tree: "one with thin foliage like hair, called easy-to-gather; another with a rugged appearance . . . and with a stronger scent . . .; and the third, tall balsam because it grows higher than the rest. The balsam from the tree with the rough bark is the choicest; that from the tall variety is next; and easy-to-gather is the lowest grade" (Pliny, *Nat. Hist.,* XII:115). He also mentions products derived from other parts of the tree, such as the xylobalsamum juice, a relatively inferior perfume produced from the branches of the balsam tree.

Strangely enough, although there are abundant historical and literary sources referring to balsam, we have no direct archaeological evidence from the Second Temple period about either its cultivation or production, only about its marketing. The only perfume of which containers bearing its name have survived is balsam. We have a store jar with the inscription *balsam balsama* on it in Aramaic and Hebrew, and a fragment, probably from another store jar, inscribed *balsaneh*, has been found at Masada. Presumably these jars contained balsam, and they may have been the "jars" that were placed in tombs: "A jar of balsam placed in the tomb and its fragrance was sweet" (*Tanhuma*, ed. Buber, 58, 6), or alternatively they may have been used for marketing the balsam. In two papyrus fragments in Latin from Masada, which have recently been deciphered, there is mention of xylobalsamum – the inferior product of the balsam tree. This find suggests that the Roman soldiers stationed in that fortress may have been involved in one way or another in the balsam trade.

A most interesting discovery is that of a Herodian pottery juglet from the 1st century CE which was recently found, wrapped in palm fibers for protection, in a cave near Qumran. The juglet contained an oily substance, whose fragrance had evaporated over the centuries. In the body of the juglet there is a round hole drilled to facilitate pouring the substance out of the vessel, and at present plugged with a small stone. The hole was meant to prevent the blocking of the narrow neck of the juglet. Chemical analysis has shown that the remaining fluid is a viscous plant oil, but not olive oil, resin, wine, or honey. Unable to identify the fluid as any known vegetable oil, scientists have suggested that it may be remains of the famous, now extinct, balsam oil.

Possible evidence of a balsam industry already in the First Temple period, has been discovered at En Gedi. Although balsam (*aparsemon*) is not mentioned in the Bible, it is usually identified with the *bosem*, a perfume-producing plant which grew in cultivated orchards: "My beloved has gone down to his garden, to the beds of spices (*bosem*), to feed in the gardens and to gather lilies" (*Song of Solomon*, 6:2). Josephus already held this view (*Ant.*, VIII:174). An early tradition cited in the Talmud links the cultivation of the balsam tree with En Gedi already during the First Temple period. According to this tradition, the "vinedressers and husbandmen" whom Nebuzaradan, Nebuchadnezzar's "captain of the guard," left behind in Judah after the destruction of the Temple (2 Kings, 25:8-12), were employed in producing balsam: " 'vinedressers'. . . – this means balsamum gatherers from En Gedi to Ramah" (Babyl. *Shabbath*, 26a). According to yet another tradition, Josiah set aside the oil of anointment, and from his time on the kings were anointed with balsam oil (Babyl. *Kerithoth*, 5b).

Excavations at En Gedi, on the western shore of the Dead Sea, have uncovered a settlement dating from the latter part of the Judaean Monarchy (7th–6th centuries BCE), with buildings and courtyards of a special character, and abounding in finds. The buildings were erected on terraces and had a spacious courtyard and two small rooms. Here the archaeologists discovered many installations and vessels that had been used for industrial purposes. Prominent among them were pottery vats about a meter high and open at the base. These were found standing in rows, one next to the other, their bases sunk into the ground, with large quantities of charcoal and ashes around them. The vats are

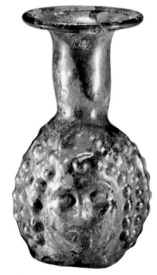

Head-vase for perfume (?),
mold-blown glass,
Eretz Israel, 4th century CE

Group of pottery vessels probably used in the perfume industry, En Gedi,
latter part of the Judaean Monarchy, late 7th–early 6th centuries BCE

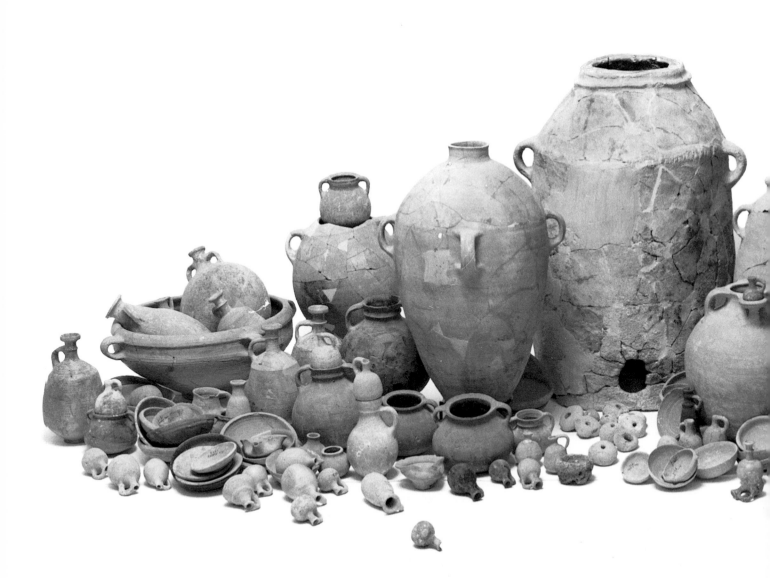

Inscription on the mosaic floor of a synagogue
at En Gedi, 6th century CE:

Remembered for good be Jose, 'Iron and Hezekio the
sons of Halfi. / Whosoever shall sow (lit. give) discord
between a man and his colleagues, or denounce / his
colleagues to the Gentiles, or steal / belongings of his
colleagues, or whosoever shall reveal the secret of the
town / to the Gentiles – May He whose eyes range
over the entire earth / and sees the hidden, He shall set
His face against that person / and his seed, and shall
uproot him from under the heavens. / And the entire
people say: Amen, amen. Selah!

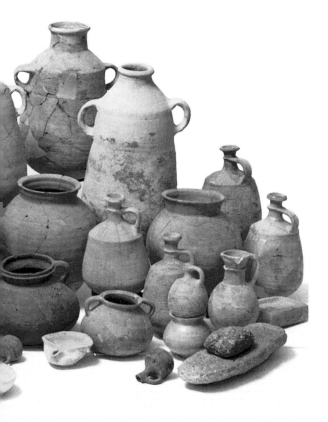

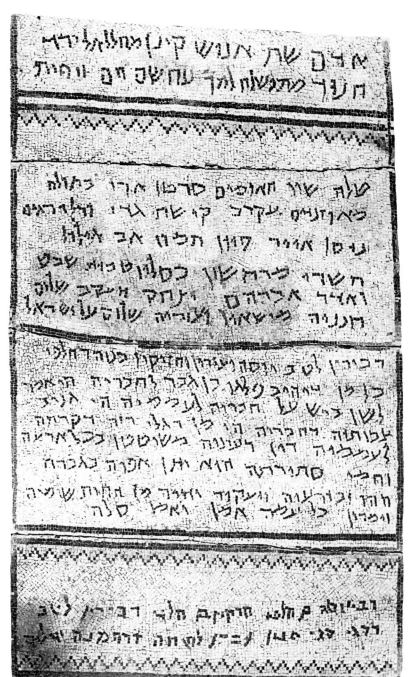

believed to have served as ovens. Several of them were surrounded with lumps of henna and perforated clay balls of various sizes. Also found in the courtyards were large pottery pithoi (storage jars), cooking pots, small bowls, jars, decanters, jugs and juglets, as well as basalt millstones. The character of the place and the assemblage of vessels attest that the work carried out there required the use of large and small as well as deep and shallow vessels, similar to kitchen equipment. The ovens and the perforated clay balls were used for heating, the storage jars probably contained oil and water, the cooking pots and kraters were used to stir the mixtures, and the jugs and decanters were suitable for holding the finished product. Comparison with other sites in the ancient East led the excavators to the conclusion that the workshop uncovered at En Gedi had produced perfumes – and what perfume would be more likely here than the balsam? If this assumption is correct, it provides some confirmation of the Talmudic tradition that since the reign of Josiah king of Judah, the oil used for the anointing of kings was balsam oil, and that the center of balsam production was at En Gedi.

As already noted, no clear archaeological traces of a balsam industry remain from the Second Temple period, either at En Gedi or anywhere else. However, a possible clue appears several hundred years later, in an unexpected source – the mosaic floor of a synagogue from the Byzantine period at En Gedi. On this floor, dating from the 6th century CE, a long inscription was discovered, containing a curse on "whoever shall reveal the secret of the town to the Gentiles." Such a forceful curse in a synagogue seems most peculiar, and the hypothesis is that the secret in question concerns the growing of balsam and the production of the perfume derived from it. What we have here, then, is probably the oath sworn by members of the En Gedi balsam-growers guild to preserve their secret.

The chain of evidence, both direct and indirect, spans many centuries. And although numerous links are missing, even without them it appears that the perfume of the Palestinian balsam was a prestigious product known throughout the ancient world, and coveted by kings and princes. What its fragrance was we may never know, but it would seem to have been irresistibly seductive. The Sages, at least, were concerned for the daughters of Jerusalem who "put myrrh and balsam in their shoes and walked through the marketplaces of Jerusalem, and on coming near to the young men of Israel . . . kicked their feet and spurted it on them, thus instilling them with passionate desire like with serpent's poison" (Babyl. *Shabbath*, 62b).

# The Spice Trade

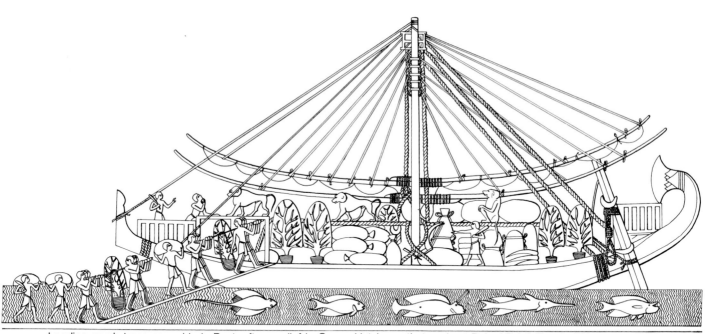

Loading myrrh trees on a ship in Punt, after a relief in Queen Hatshepsut's temple at Deir el-Bahri, Egypt, 15th century BCE

The wide use of perfumes and spices in the ancient East created a great demand for them, and thus an extensive trade developed in these products. From Assyrian sources, the Bible, as well as from classical authors, it appears that the center of the trade in aromatic resins and incense was located in the kingdoms of South Arabia, where some of these precious aromatics were grown. From there major land and sea trade routes led to all the great centers of the ancient world. An important role in the marketing of perfumes and spices was played by the Nabataeans, who functioned as middlemen; Palestine too had an important share, especially in the transportation of these goods to the Mediterranean coast and further west.

Since perfume products were so essential and so difficult to obtain, the kings of Egypt and Mesopotamia had already tried to import trees and seedlings to enable them to grow and produce spices and incense in their own countries. It is known that the Egyptian Queen Hatshepsut, who lived in the first half of the 15th century BCE, sent a royal expedition consisting of five ships to the land of Punt (Somalia), in order to bring back myrrh and myrrh seedlings to plant in her temple. This voyage is commemorated in inscriptions and reliefs on the walls of her temple at Deir el-Bahri. But it appears that the seedlings did not take well in Egypt, possibly because they were of inferior quality, or because they were damaged when they were dug up, or perhaps because of some action taken by the people of Punt to protect their economic interests and the lucrative Egyptian market for their products. When Egypt's power declined, in the last quarter of the 2nd millennium BCE, the expeditions to Punt ceased, but the demand for spices did not diminish, and so the Egyptians turned eastward, to Arabia, and imported myrrh and frankincense from there on camelback, by the desert routes. In Assyrian records of tribute and spoils of war, perfumes and resins are mentioned, and a text from the time of Tukulti-Ninurta II (890–884 BCE) refers to balls of myrrh among the tribute brought to the Assyrian king by the Aramaean kingdoms.

Most of the spices and incense-producing plants came from the Far East, and especially from South Arabia, as mentioned by Isaiah, 60:6: "A multitude of camels shall cover you . . . all those from Sheba shall come, they shall bring gold and frankincense." Of the Queen of Sheba, whose kingdom was in South Arabia, it is told that when she came to Jerusalem to visit King Solomon, she brought "camels bearing spices" (1 Kings, 10:2). It may well be that during Solomon's reign the Kingdom of Israel had taken over Egypt's traditional role of safeguarding the spice caravans passing through Palestine. It is also possible that the numerous fortresses that were built in the Negev during this period, dated by some scholars to the 10th century BCE, the time of King Solomon's reign, are connected to the control of the caravan routes. Arabia is also mentioned as the source of the spices in the trade with the Kingdom of Tyre (Ezekiel, 27:22).

The trade relations between Palestine and South Arabia may be reflected by potsherds of the 7th–6th centuries BCE bearing incised signs in South Arabian script that have been

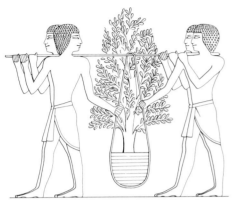

Myrrh seedling being taken to Egypt, after a relief in Queen Hatshepsut's temple at Deir el-Bahri, Egypt, 15th century BCE

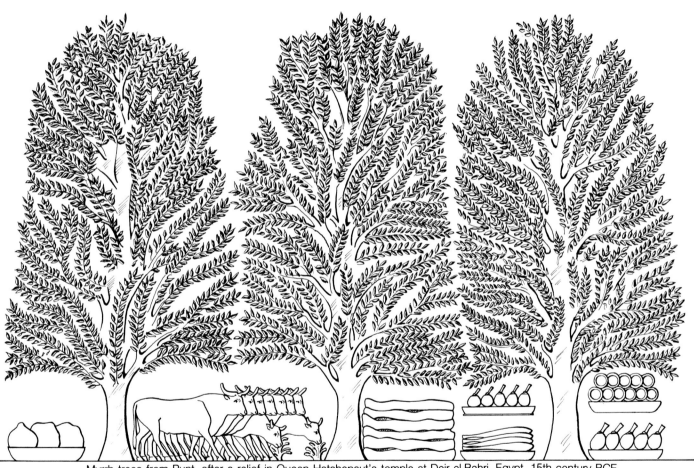

Myrrh trees from Punt, after a relief in Queen Hatshepsut's temple at Deir el-Bahri, Egypt, 15th century BCE

found at various sites, including the City of David in Jerusalem, and Tell el-Kheleifeh, near modern Eilat. Two ostraca (potsherds) bearing South Arabian signs from the 4th–3rd centuries BCE were discovered at Tell Jemmeh. Written in ink on one of these is *ABM*, a name that also appears in other South Arabian inscriptions found along the "incense route" in Arabia. Some authorities see this as evidence of the passage of a camel caravan carrying myrrh and frankincense from South Arabia to the port of Gaza. The inscriptions found in Jerusalem are certainly also connected with the spice trade, since large quantities of spices for incense, especially frankincense, were used in the Temple. These inscriptions were found on locally made vessels, perhaps indicating that on their return journeys the caravans took equipment from Jerusalem, or barter for the goods they had brought.

This is the place to mention a broken clay stamp found in the excavations at Bethel, bearing the South Arabian name "Hamiyan the delegate" in South Arabian script. The stamp was dated to the 9th century BCE, as a result of historical considerations, and because of its shape and size (7 x 8 cm), the excavators believed that it had served to seal bags made of leather or fabric, which were suitable for packing spice plants or resin, and hence considered it evidence of incense supply to the shrine at Bethel. According to another opinion, however, this stamp originated in Hadhramaut, and got to Bethel by chance, in modern times.

Most of the spices and perfume plants were brought from distant lands: cinnamon from Ceylon and China; aloes, produced from a tropical tree, from India; spikenard, which was one of the costliest perfumes, from Nepal and the Himalayas. However, the spice trade centered mainly on myrrh and frankincense, which grew in South Arabia and North Somalia. These two substances were consumed in the greatest quantities, since they served as incense for ritual and domestic purposes as well as for funerary practices, medicine and cosmetics.

Myrrh was used mainly for perfumes and cosmetics, as recounted in the Book of Esther: "for so were the days of their beautifying accomplished: six months with oil of myrrh" (2:12), but it was also an ingredient in medicines, and in Egypt it was used in embalming. In the Bible it is frequently mentioned as one of the constituents of the incense in the Temple, and Plutarch also refers to it, in this context, with regard to Egypt in the classical period (*Isis and Osiris*, 52).

Frankincense, too, was used for cosmetics and perfumes, as well as for medical purposes – to stanch bleeding, heal wounds, and the like. It was one of the four ingredients of the incense used in the Tabernacle (Exodus, 30:34), and was kept with the Temple treasures (1 Chronicles, 9:29). It was also commonly used for domestic incense, and was presumably burned on the small incense altars made of stone and pottery, some of them inscribed with names of spices, which were prevalent mainly between the 6th and the

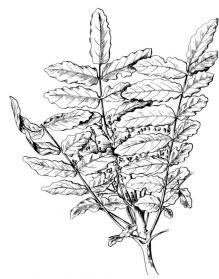

Branch of the frankincense shrub

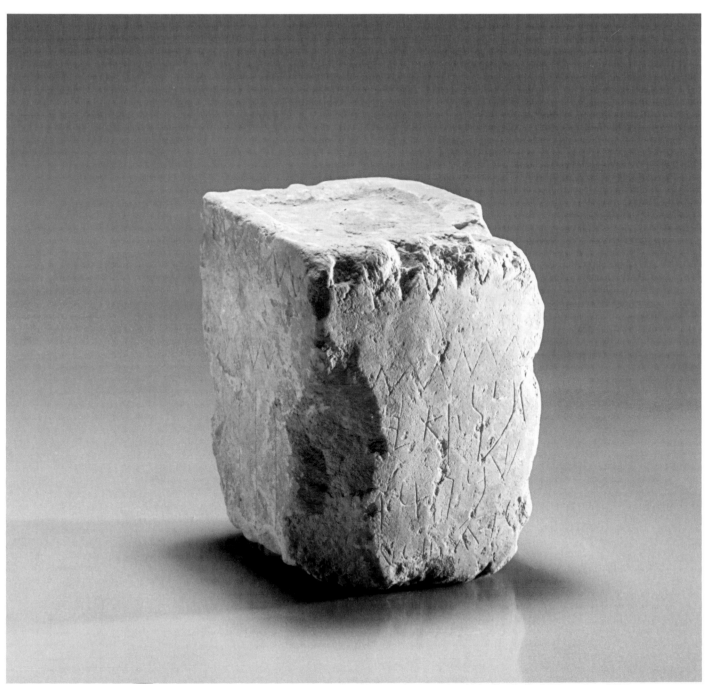

Small incense altar, incised with the word lebonta (frankincense), stone, Lachish, first half of 5th century BCE

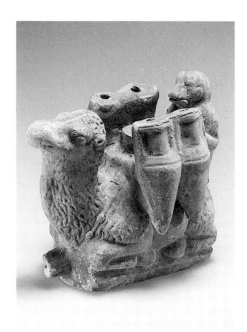

Camel carrying jars, pottery figurine, Roman period

4th centuries BCE. At Lachish a small stone incense altar has been uncovered, bearing the incised word *lebonta* (frankincense in Aramaic). The chief use of frankincense, however, was in cremation burials, both to propitiate the gods and to overcome the stench of the burning bodies. Pliny reports that at the cremation of Nero's wife Poppaea, a full year's production of frankincense was burned on her funeral pyre (*Nat. Hist.*, XII: 83).

Frankincense grew mainly in the southeastern region of the Arabian peninsula, in the mountains of Dhofar, a journey of eight days from Sabota (Shabwa), the capital of Hadhramaut. The frankincense plant is a shrub with low branches and produces a transparent yellowish resin, from which the aromatic essence is obtained. The myrrh tree, in contrast, which grew in Southwest Arabia and in North Somalia, is tall and has a reddish-brown resin. The resin was generally gathered from the trees in the summer, but during the Roman period, with the increased demand for perfume, a second yield was obtained from the trees in early spring. Towards winter, at the end of the gathering, the gum-resin was prepared for shipment: the myrrh was packed in leather bags, to preserve its oily constituent, while the frankincense, a dry substance, was packed in baskets with the greatest care, so as not to crush the "teardrops" of resin or break the branches (Pliny, *Nat. Hist.*, XII:52–71). Of these organic packing materials no trace has survived.

The increasing demand for spices, especially for myrrh and frankincense, led to the development of an extensive network of trade-routes, by land, by sea, or by combinations of both, connecting East to West, India and Arabia to Mesopotamia, Syria, Palestine, Egypt, Greece, and Rome. Overland transportation was mainly on camel-back. The camel was domesticated in the 13th–12th centuries BCE, and from then on became an important means of transportation linking the Arabian peninsula with countries of the Fertile Crescent.

Overland transportation followed several different routes, corresponding to the rise and fall of the various South Arabian kingdoms. The principal overland route from South Arabia to the Fertile Crescent – known as "the incense route" – went north along the west side of the Arabian peninsula, parallel to the Red Sea. It has been suggested that this route may already have been in existence in the 10th century BCE, and that the Queen of Sheba traveled along it on her journey to Jerusalem.

This route began at Shabwa, and along it there were 65 stopping stations, among them Timna, Marib, Ma'in, Yathrib, Dedan and Gaza (Pliny, *Nat. Hist.*, XII:65). At its end, the route divided into several branches. One led to Eilat and to Palestine, or to Sinai and Egypt, another to the port of Leuce Come, on the east shore of the Red Sea, and from there by land to Petra and Damascus. One route branched off at Teima to Mesopotamia. Yet another overland route crossed the Arabian peninsula from Wadi Hadhramaut and turned east to the Gerrha region, near the Persian Gulf, a journey of 40 days. From there the frankincense was shipped to Mesopotamia and Palestine (Strabo, *Geography*, XVI:3.3; 4.4).

Map of routes in the spice and perfume trade

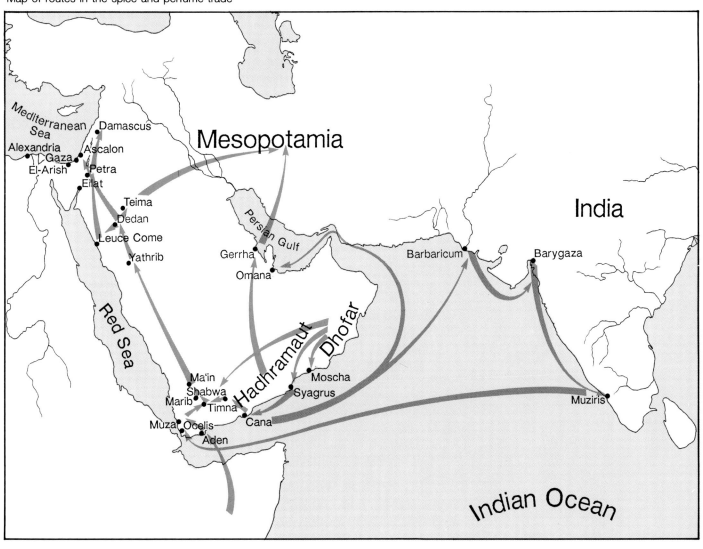

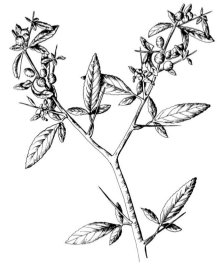

Myrrh branch

Transportation by sea gained great momentum after the regularity of the monsoon winds was discovered in the 1st century BCE by the Greek seafarer Hippalus. From then on it became possible to sail along the eastern coast of Africa and to reach India by sea.

Frankincense was transported from the forests in Dhofar to the ports of Moscha and Syagrus in South Arabia, and from there it was shipped on during the winter – part of it to Cana, the principal port of Hadhramaut, and part to Egypt. From Cana, some of it was sent north to Shabwa and the rest was stored until the following summer, for transportation to India. Frankincense that was not sent by sea was transported overland from Dhofar to Shabwa.

Another frankincense sea-route went east from the port of Cana to the Persian Gulf, where the frankincense ships called at several ports, Omana among them. Other sea-routes went to Northwest India, where the frankincense ships called at Barbaricum and Barygaza, and to Southwest India, where they anchored at the port of Muziris. On their way back from India the ships set out during the winter months, to exploit the northeast monsoon winds, and sailed to the port of Ocelis. But if they were delayed in departure they sailed to Moscha, where they wintered, continuing on to Egypt only when the weather improved. The myrrh was transported from Southwest Arabia and Somalia to the ports of Aden and Muza and from there to Timna and Shabwa.

The South Arabian kingdoms' monopoly of the growth and production of incense plants and their control of transportation and trade routes brought them great wealth, so much so that in the first century CE the Arabians were considered the wealthiest race in the world (Pliny, *Nat. Hist.*, VI:161).

An important role in the spice and incense trade between South Arabia and the Mediterranean coast was played by the Nabataeans. They were the intermediaries in the transportation of the spices that came by sea from India and the Far East to the ports of South Arabia, and from there to the Nabataean centers in North Arabia. They also established a system of waystations along the trade routes leading from Leuce Come in the north of the Arabian peninsula to Petra and Damascus. The Nabataean control of this trade reached its peak at some time between the later part of the 1st century BCE and the mid-1st century CE. The great wealth the Nabataeans accumulated in this way is described in the works of Diodorus Siculus, who lived in the 1st century BCE: "While there are many Arabian tribes who use the desert as pasture, the Nabataeans far surpass the others in wealth, although they are not much more than ten thousand in number; for not a few of them are accustomed to bring down to the sea frankincense and myrrh and the most valuable kinds of spices, which they procure . . . from what is called Arabia Felix" (Diodorus Siculus, XIX:94, 5).

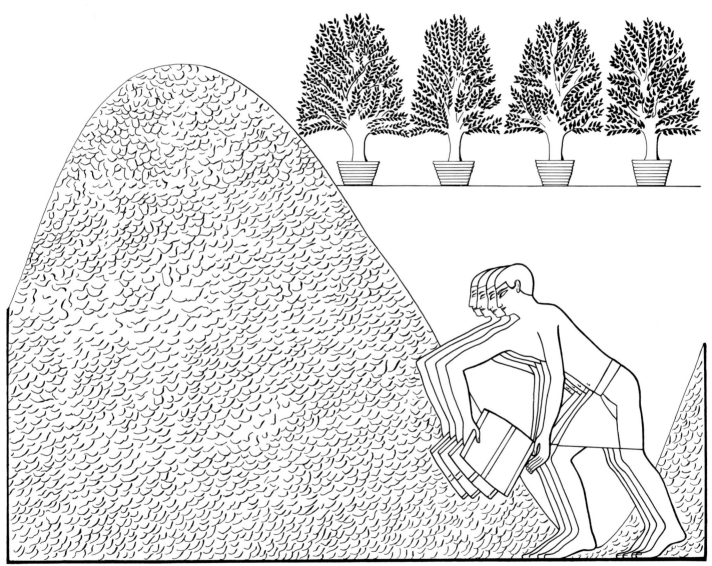

Workers filling containers with myrrh extracted from the tree, after a relief in Queen Hatshepsut's temple, Deir el-Bahri, Egypt, 15th century BCE

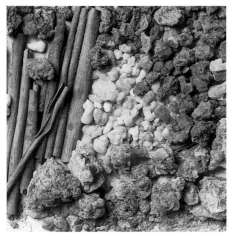

Myrrh, frankincense, cinnamon, and resin

An important trade route connected Petra to Gaza from late in the 4th century BCE to the mid-1st century CE, and contributed greatly to Gaza's prosperity. The port of Gaza became an important export center for goods from South Arabia to the Western Mediterranean (Pliny, *Nat. Hist.*, XII:65).

Interesting details about Gaza in the 3rd century BCE have been found in the papyri of Zenon, a high official in the service of Apollonius, treasurer to Ptolemy II. In his time an officer was in charge of the incense trade passing through Gaza. Besides Gaza, the ports of Ascalon and el-Arish benefited from the spice trade.

Although all these trade routes were well established, the transportation of perfumes and spices was still long and hazardous. Many dangers lurked along the desert routes for the spice caravans, and for the ships there were the various perils of the sea, pirates among them. In addition, heavy taxes were imposed on carriers of spices, especially on the overland caravans, as Pliny records: "Fixed portions of frankincense are also given to the priests and the king's secretaries, but beside these the guards and their attendants and the gate-keepers and servants also have their pickings. Indeed, all along the route they keep on paying, at one place for water, at another for fodder or the charges for lodging at the halts and the various octrois. So that expenses mount up to 688 denarii per camel before the Mediterranean coast is reached" (Pliny, *Nat. Hist.*, XII:65).

It is no wonder that under such conditions, the prices of perfumes and spices soared to exceeding heights. The great demand for them, together with the limited supply, also made them a target for thieves, even during the processing stage, and thus strict security measures had to be taken to guard them: "At Alexandria . . . where the frankincense is worked up for sale . . . a seal is put upon the workmen's aprons, they have to wear a mask . . . and before they are allowed to leave the premises they have to take off all their clothes" (Pliny, *Nat. Hist.*, XII:59).

Commercial relations between the ends of the world, as it was known then, reached their peak during the 2nd century CE, when the Romans succeeded in sailing directly to the sources of the perfumes and spices in South Arabia and India, and as a result the South Arabian kingdoms declined in importance. From the 4th century on, when Christianity became the official religion, the practice of cremation was ceased, and the return to ordinary burial led to a great decrease in the use of incense. The consumption of cosmetics for personal beautification also declined drastically in the Christian world, which frowned on luxuriousness and indulgence in bodily pleasures. Trade in spices and resins used for the cosmetics industry and for medical purposes did not cease, but the quantities consumed from then on were negligible when compared to those used previously, and thus the perfume trade began to die out.

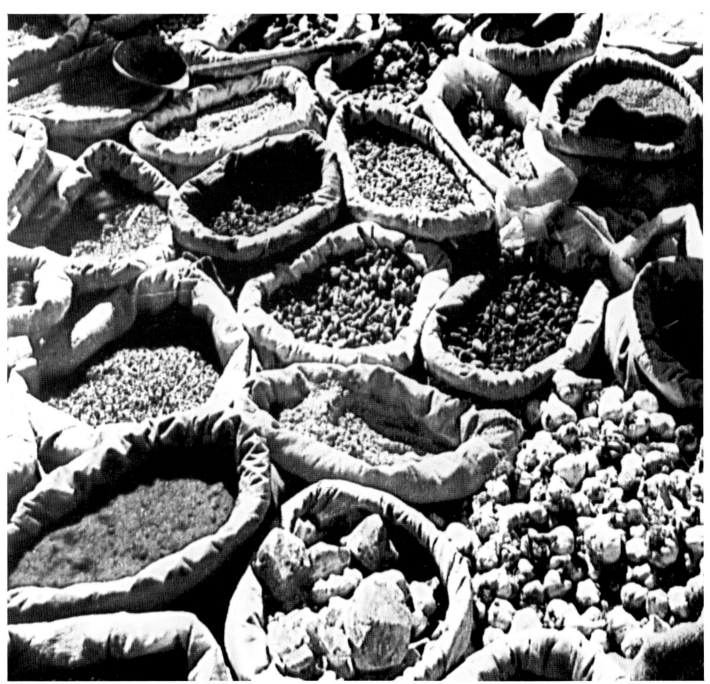

Selected spices in sacks

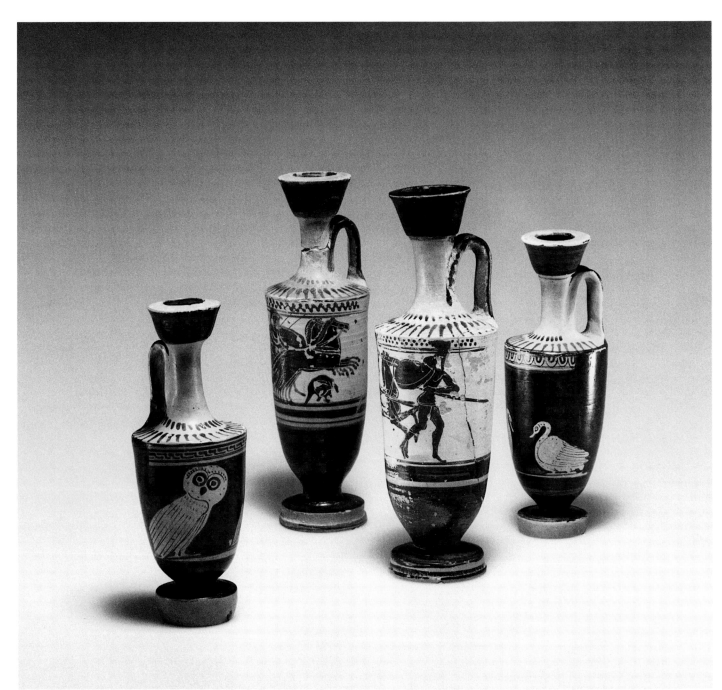

Lekythoi, Greece, 6th–5th centuries BCE

# Spices in Funerary Customs

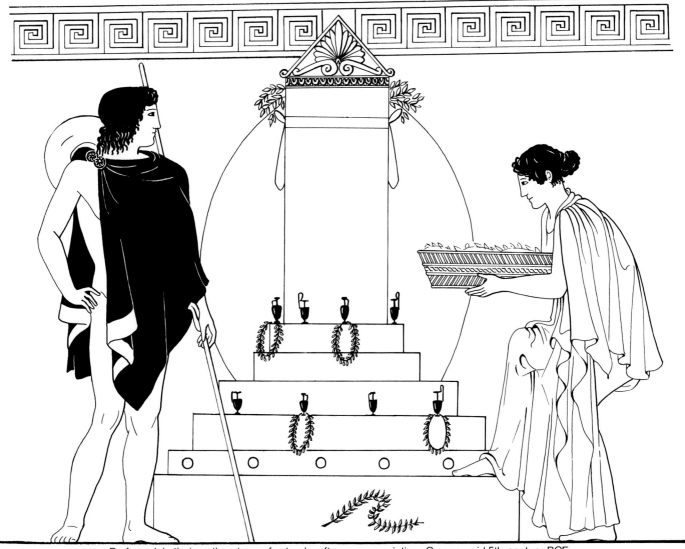

Perfume lekythoi on the steps of a tomb, after a vase painting, Greece, mid-5th century BCE

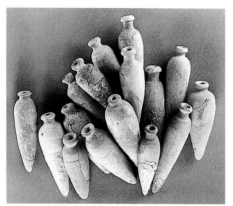

Carrot-shaped perfume bottles from burial caves at Ketef Hinnom, Jerusalem, 6th–5th centuries BCE

In antiquity, burial and burial customs held a central place in people's consciousness, for man's last resting place was conceived as a continuation of his earthly life. To make the deceased person's passage to the afterlife more pleasant, he was buried with some of his personal belongings, and was equipped with food, drink, and offerings. Included among the latter was an assortment of toilet articles, ointments and perfumes. We will discuss these burial customs in the light of tombs of the First and Second Temple periods in Eretz Israel, though they were common and widespread in all the cultures of the ancient world.

The funerary gifts were intended to give the deceased a sense of his accustomed environment. In Egypt, this practice attained outstanding forms of expression: there the tombs contained an abundance of objects, including a variety of aromatic oils and ointments. The functions of these ointments are described in a chapter of the *Book of the Dead*, which deals with the preparation of the body for burial. The Egyptians also ornamented the walls of the tombs with reliefs and paintings depicting scenes from the daily life of the deceased. These pictures were believed to exert a magical influence and preserve the deceased's prior status. The funerary gifts had to be renewed regularly, an obligation that was placed upon the deceased's son or on the priests responsible for the mortuary ritual. Our knowledge about Egyptian burial customs draws mainly on tombs of kings and nobles as well as on the *Book of the Dead*, which contained instructions and guidance concerning life in the netherworld.

In Eretz Israel during the First Temple period, a person's burial place was conceived as a continuation of his dwelling in the world of the living. The Israelite was usually buried in a tomb which one of his ancestors had acquired several generations earlier, and which had been used since then as a family tomb (Genesis, 49:29). From the Bible little can be gleaned about forms of burial or burial rites current among the Israelites, but some passages refer to mourning customs and matters of defilement and purity (Numbers, 19:14–19). The usual tomb of this period was hewn into the rock; at times a natural cave was adapted for this purpose. Such a tomb contained a single burial chamber, though in the course of time more chambers were added to accomodate new burials. Around the walls of the chamber benches were hewn for the bodies of the deceased and their grave goods – personal belongings, pottery vessels, cosmetic containers, jewelry, and other artifacts. Since these family tombs continued to be used over several generations, it became necessary to make room for the newly deceased by collecting the bones of those previously buried, together with their funerary offerings, and placing them in one of the corners of the chamber, or in a rock-cut repository underneath the chamber. This space-saving method made it possible for several generations of a family or clan to be buried in the same tomb. From this custom comes the concept of "the Tomb of the Fathers." At times such a tomb went out of use, and after an interval of some decades or even centuries, it would be reopened, most probably to be used by a different family.

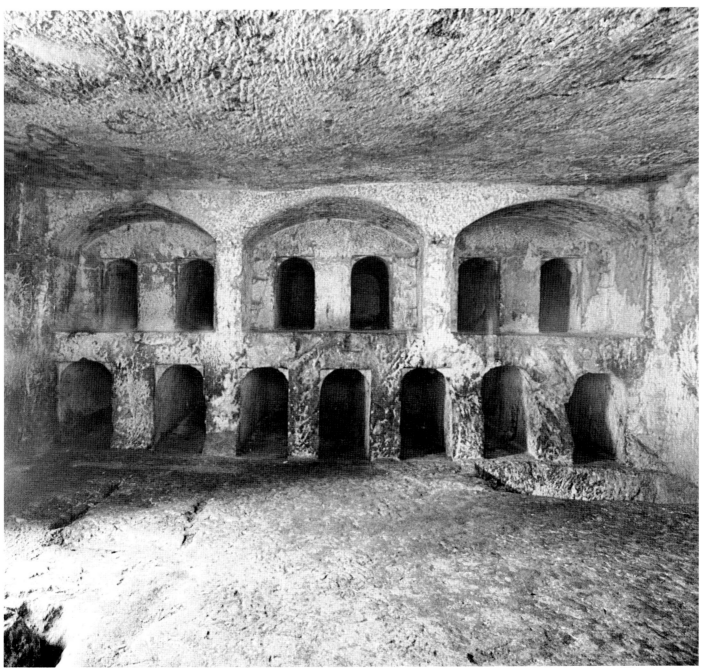

Characteristic burial cave of the Second Temple period, Sanhedriya, Jerusalem, 1st century BCE–1st century CE

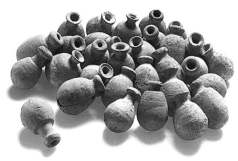

Spherical perfume bottles from burial caves at Ketef Hinnom, Jerusalem, 6th–5th centuries BCE

Most of the burial caves of the First Temple period that have been uncovered date from the latter part of the Judaean Monarchy, and the majority have been found in Jerusalem, though some were discovered at other sites. Most of the tombs had suffered pillage and destruction at the hands of tomb-robbers and only seldom did some of the grave-goods escape the plunderers' eyes. One of the most important of these tombs is a burial cave discovered at Ketef Hinnom in Jerusalem, dating from the 7th–6th centuries BCE. Here the repository, with all its original contents, has been preserved, although the burial chamber itself had been pillaged and was found empty. Among the finds recovered in the repository were pottery oil-lamps, decanter jugs, and perfume bottles in large numbers, as well as the famous silver amulets inscribed with the Priestly Benediction. Similar assemblages of vessels, though smaller, have been found in other tombs of the period. It is noteworthy that in contrast to tombs of earlier periods, which contained many vessels for cooking and eating, in the tombs of the 7th–6th centuries BCE cooking and storage vessels are absent, while perfume bottles, lamps, and decanters are prominently represented. Presumably, these were connected with the preparation of the body for burial or with the burial rites. The biblical verses describing the burial of King Asa of Judah mention the use of perfumes and spices: "They buried him in his own sepulchers which he had hewed out for himself in the City of David. They laid him on a bier which was filled with sweet odors and various kinds of spices; and they made a very great burning for him" (2 Chronicles, 16:14). Perhaps this passage can be interpreted as some indication of changes in conceptions and beliefs concerning life after death.

The tombs of the Second Temple period were mostly burial caves, which to some extent continued the traditions of the First Temple period. Here, too, we find the practice of rock-cut family tombs which were used for several generations. The tombs contained a burial chamber with niches (*kokhim*), into which the deceased were laid. In the next stage, probably about a year later, after the flesh had decomposed, family members or friends collected the bones of the deceased (Mishnah *Sanhedrin*, 6:6), and placed them in an ossuary (stone box). Generally, the bones of only one person were put in the ossuary, but at times the bones of close relatives were added. Bone collection was practiced mainly in Jerusalem and its surroundings, where more than two thousand ossuaries have been found. The earliest evidence of this practice is from the time of Herod the Great, in the last quarter of the 1st century BCE, and it is known to have been connected with new concepts of individual resurrection, the origins of which can be traced to an earlier period (Daniel, 12:2; 2 Maccabees, 7:9–23; 12:43–44). After the destruction of the Temple, this practice gradually disappeared, though a few instances are known until as late as the early 3rd century CE.

Our knowledge of burial customs during the First Temple period is based mainly on archaeological evidence, but as regards the Second Temple period we have abundant written sources in addition to the archaeological material. Extensive discussions of burials and burial practices occur in Mishnaic and Talmudic literature, and the large numbers of

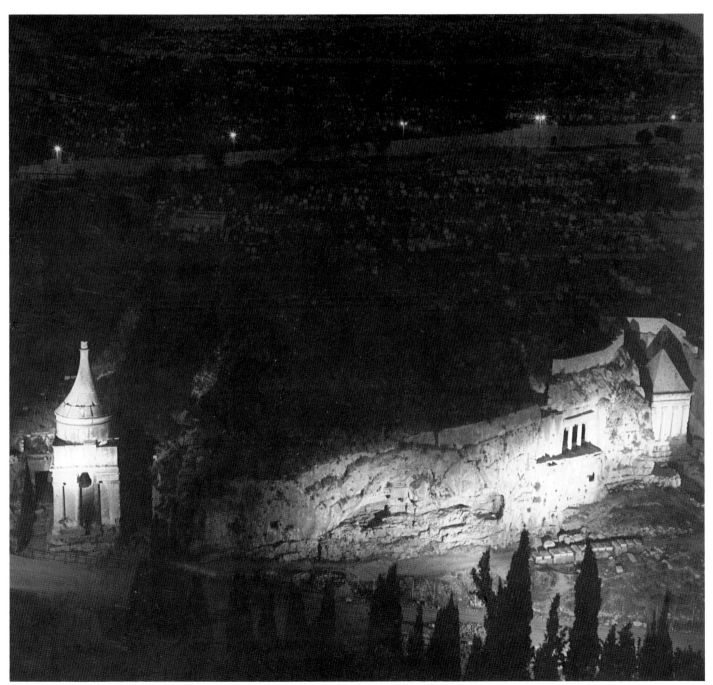

Funerary monuments, Qidron Valley, Jerusalem

burial caves that have survived from the period further elucidate the subject. Funerary offerings have also been found in tombs of the Second Temple and Talmudic periods. Usually, these are scattered in various parts of the tomb, rather than next to the bodies in the *kokhim* or in the ossuaries. Hence it is difficult to determine whether these were personal belongings, placed in the tomb in honor of the deceased, or whether they had been brought by the mourners. There are some indications in the sources that these vessels belonged either to those in charge of the burial and were used in the preparation of the body for primary or secondary burial, or were brought there by the mourners. It is known, for instance, that during the primary burial perfumes were sprinkled before the bier (Tosefta *Shekalim*, 1:12). In the Mishnah we read that the body was anointed and washed, which means that it was cleaned with oil and washed with water before being wrapped in a shroud (*Shabbath*, 23:5). The washing and anointing were performed by relatives and friends in the house of the deceased or in the place where he died (*Semahot*, 1:3). The practice of anointing the body of the deceased with aromatic oils is also mentioned in the New Testament: "And when the Sabbath was past, Mary Magdalene and Mary the mother of James, and Salome, had bought sweet spices, that they might come and anoint him" (Mark, 16:1); "And there came also Nicodemus, which at first came to Jesus by night, and brought a mixture of myrrh and aloes, about a hundred pound weight. Then they took the body of Jesus, and wound it in linen clothes with the spices, as the manner of the Jews is to bury" (John, 19:39–40).

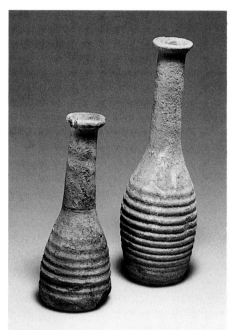

Ribbed bottles for oil or perfume from tombs, pottery, Eretz Israel, Late Roman period

The numerous bottles and juglets which had contained the spices and oils used in these rites were placed next to the body, and sometimes they were removed, together with the collected bones of the deceased, for secondary burial. In this connection it is of interest that in many cases black or brown stains have been found on the bones in the ossuaries. Presumably, these are traces of the oils that were sprinkled on the bones at the time of the secondary burial. This practice of sprinkling oil or wine on the bones is mentioned in the Mishnah: "The bones may be sprinkled with wine and oil. So Rabbi Akiba. Rabbi Simeon ben Nannas says: oil, but not wine, because wine evaporates. Neither wine nor oil, say the Sages, because these only invite worms, but dried herbs may be put on them" (*Semahot*, 12:9).

Bottles and juglets, as already mentioned, are frequently found among the funerary offerings, and many of them must have contained spices or oils. A hint of the presence of spices in tombs is found in the Mishnaic prohibition: "No benediction may be said over . . . spices used for the dead" (*Berakhot*, 8:6). They are also mentioned in the Talmud: "The spices are to remove the bad smell" (Babyl. *Berakhot*, 53a).

The "spices of the dead" included some of the most famous fragrances of the ancient world, such as the *aparsemon* (balsam): "A jug of balsam which was placed in the tomb gave off a good smell" (*Tanhuma*, ed. Buber, 58:6), and also "A flask of foliatum (an oil

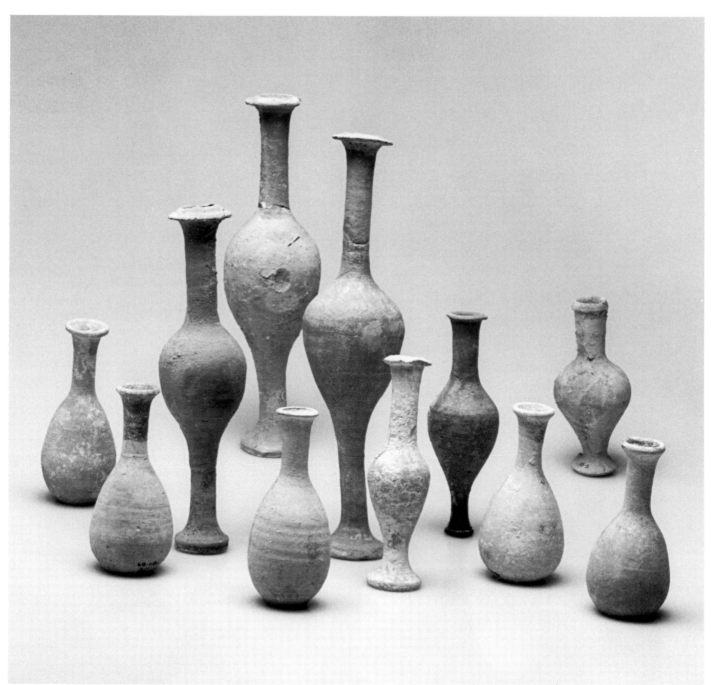

Spindle- and pear-shaped bottles, pottery, Eretz Israel, late 2nd century BCE–1st century CE

prepared from leaves of spikenard) . . . stood in the cemetery and its smell was spreading" (*Yalqut Shimoni*, Gen., 49; see chapter on "Perfume Production").

The practice of sprinkling the body of the dead with aromatic spices can be understood against the background of the country's warm climate. The spices were intended to slow down the process of decomposition and to repel flies and insects. However, they were intended not only for the deceased, as part of the burial rites, but also for the place of burial itself. There is no doubt that many of the bottles that have been found were brought by the mourners, in order to mitigate the bad smell and to freshen the air during and after the burial ceremony. This was certainly a necessary procedure in family tombs, which were visited at set times.

The practice of placing bottles of perfume beside the dead was also prevalent in classical Greece. There, too, it was customary to wash the body and then anoint it with oil. This work was generally carried out by female relatives of the deceased. The most common perfume bottle was the white-ground lekythos, often decorated with funerary scenes. Sometimes these vessels had false interior chambers so that they should hold only a small quantity of precious liquid. It was customary to place them around the bier, and in funerary scenes they are often seen standing on the steps of the tombstone or hanging from it. In Roman tombs, too, fragrant oils played an important part in funerary practices, and large quantities of spices and incense were used at cremations. Royal burials naturally required especially large quantities of spices. Josephus recounts that at King Herod's funeral, "five hundred servants carrying spices" walked behind his coffin (*Ant.*, 17:199), and in describing the funeral of Aristobulus, Josephus mentions "a great quantity of spices" (*ibid.*, 15:61).

The numerous bottles found in the tombs complement the written sources. It is interesting to note that many of the bottles found are of poor quality and carelessly manufactured, possibly because they were made especially for funerary use. Towards the end of the First Temple period, the alabastron begins to appear in tombs, together with carrot-shaped, spherical, and pear-shaped bottles. The alabastron was common between the 7th and 5th centuries BCE, especially during the 6th century, and is an imitation of the Egyptian alabaster bottles that were prevalent during the Persian period. The carrot-shaped bottles were current from the 6th to the 4th centuries BCE, and imitate an Assyrian prototype. The spherical bottle also derived from an Assyrian prototype, and was fairly common during the Persian period. Characteristic of all these three types is their rounded or pointed base, which does not allow them to be stood upright without support – a feature not needed in the tombs.

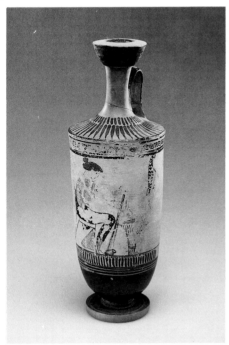

Lekythos for perfume, pottery, Greece, 5th century BCE

In tombs of the Hellenistic period, the spindle-shaped bottle was particularly prevalent. This type of bottle originated in the Western Mediterranean area in the 4th century BCE, while in Palestine it became highly popular in the late 2nd and early 1st centuries BCE. It apparently replaced the lekythos of classical times. The spindle-shaped bottle was gradually supplanted by the pear-shaped bottle, which began to appear in the second half of the 1st century BCE and was particularly popular until the destruction of the Second Temple. This type of bottle had several advantages over its predecessor, being lighter and more stable. Another type, the so-called candlestick bottle, is made of glass and has a long, narrow neck. Such bottles, known mainly from tombs, have been found in great quantities, sometimes numbering several dozens in a single tomb. Nineteenth-century scholars believed them to be tear-receptacles placed by the mourners in the tombs of their dear ones, and called them *lacrimatoria*, or "tear-bottles." Today, however, they are thought to have contained oil or perfume, and sediment-tests from two bottles of this type from the Jerusalem area have indeed shown that they contained traces of olive oil (see chapter on "Perfume Production").

## Ownership Credits

p. 16:
Inscribed vessel, Galerie Nefer, Zurich

p. 17:
Private collection

p. 21:
Private collection

p. 22:
Israel Department of Antiquities and
Museums

p. 23:
Second from right: Jonathan Rosen
Collection, New York
All others: Leo Mildenberg Collection, Zurich

p. 24:
Right: Israel Department of Antiquities and
Museums
Middle and left: Bible Lands Museum,
Jerusalem (Elie Borowski Collection)

p. 25:
Israel Department of Antiquities and
Museums

p. 26:
Private collection

p. 27:
Second from left: Bible Lands Museum,
Jerusalem (Elie Borowski Collection)

p. 28:
Right: Israel Department of Antiquities and
Museums

p. 29:
Israel Department of Antiquities and
Museums

p. 30:
Reuben and Edith Hecht Museum, University
of Haifa, Haifa

p. 31:
Below: Israel Department of Antiquities and
Museums

pp. 32, 37:
Galerie Nefer, Zurich

p. 41:
Below left: Private collection

p. 42:
Eretz Israel Museum, Tel Aviv

p. 43:
Bible Lands Museum, Jerusalem
(Elie Borowski Collection)

p. 44:
Galerie Nefer, Zurich

p. 45:
Below: Israel Department of Antiquities and
Museums

p. 47:
Second from left: Galerie Nefer, Zurich
All others: Jonathan Rosen Collection,
New York

p. 48:
Right: Private collection
Left: Israel Department of Antiquities and
Museums

p. 50:
Private collection

p. 51:
Israel Department of Antiquities and
Museums

p. 53:
Bible Lands Museum, Jerusalem
(Elie Borowski Collection)

p. 54:
Private collection

p. 63:
Galerie Nefer, Zurich

pp. 70–71:
Bible Lands Museum, Jerusalem
(Elie Borowski Collection)

p. 73:
Israel Department of Antiquities and
Museums

pp. 78, 80–81:
Israel Department of Antiquities and
Museums

p. 82:
Private collection

p. 84:
Private collection

pp. 86–88:
Israel Department of Antiquities and
Museums

p. 99
Front four: Israel Department of Antiquities and
Museums

pp. 100–102:
Israel Department of Antiquities and
Museums

p. 103:
Elie Borowski Collection, Toronto

## Ownership Credits

pp. 104–105:
Israel Department of Antiquities and Museums

p. 107:
Archaeological Staff Officer of Judaea and Samaria

pp. 109–117:
Israel Department of Antiquities and Museums

p. 118:
Eretz Israel Museum, Tel Aviv

p. 124:
Far right and left: Leo Mildenberg Collection, Zurich

pp. 126, 128:
Israel Department of Antiquities and Museums, courtesy of G. Barkay, Ketef Hinnom Expedition

pp. 130–131:
Israel Department of Antiquities and Museums

p. 132:
Museum of Regional and Mediterranean Archaeology, Gan Hashlosha

All other items belong to the Israel Museum Collection

## List of Illustrations

Photographs from books and catalogues are reproduced by courtesy of the publishers.

p. 1: after
Ch. Daremberg, E. Saglio et E. Pottier, *Dictionnaire des Antiquités grecques et romaines*, V, Hachette, Paris 1874–1919, s.v. "Unguentum," p. 594, fig. 7233. Henceforth: Daremberg

p. 7: after
J.G. Wilkinson, *The Manners and Customs of the Ancient Egyptians*, II, London 1878, p. 353, fig. 458. Henceforth: Wilkinson

p. 9: after
*Egypt's Golden Age: The Art of Living in the New Kingdom 1558–1058 B.C.,* Museum of Fine Arts, Boston 1982, p. 199, fig. 52. Henceforth: *Egypt's Golden Age*

p. 10: after
A. Erman, *Life in Ancient Egypt,* Dover Publications Inc., New York 1971, p. 214. Henceforth: Erman

p. 13: after
Daremberg, I, s.v. "Balneum," p. 650, fig. 746.

p. 18: after
Gisela M.A. Richter & Marjorie J. Milne, *Shapes and Names of Athenian Vases,* The Metropolitan Museum of Art, New York 1935, p. 16. Henceforth: Richter & Milne

p. 19: after
Richter & Milne, p. 21.

p. 33: after
Daremberg, I, s.v. "Balneum," p. 649, fig. 745.

p. 35: after
*Egypt's Golden Age,* p. 230.

p. 36: after
R.J. Forbes, *Studies in Ancient Technology,* III, rev. ed., E.J. Brill, Leiden 1965, p. 20, fig. 4. Henceforth: Forbes

p. 38: after
*Egypt's Golden Age,* p. 216, fig. 57.

p. 52: after
K. Lange & M. Hirmer, *Ägypten,* Hirmer Verlag, München 1967, pl. XXII. Henceforth: Lange & Hirmer

p. 55: after
A. Maiuri, *Roman Painting,* Skira, Geneva 1953, p. 100. Henceforth: Maiuri

p. 56: after
Lange & Hirmer, pl. XXIII.

p. 57: after
Lange & Hirmer, pl. XXXVII.

p. 59: after
Forbes, p. 21, fig. 5.

p. 60: after
Wilkinson, p. 339, fig. 446.

p. 61: after
Lange & Hirmer, fig. 205.

p. 62: after
Lange & Hirmer, fig. 176.

p. 64: after
*Egypt's Golden Age,* p. 190, fig. 49.

p. 65: after
Lange & Hirmer, fig. 56.

p. 66 above: after
M. Gauthier-Laurent, *Les Scènes de Coiffure Féminine dans L'Ancienne Egypte,* in *Melanges Maspero* I, Imprimerie de l'Institut Français d'Archéologie Orientale, le Caire 1935–38, p. 689, fig. 9. Henceforth: Gauthier-Laurent

p. 66 below: after
T.A. Madhloom, *The Chronology of Neo-Assyrian Art,* University of London, The Athlone Press, London 1970, pl. LXVI.

p. 67: after
Gauthier-Laurent, p. 677, fig. 3.

p. 68:
*Encyclopédie Photographique de L'Art* 8 (1935), pl. 238.

p. 72: after
D. Ussishkin, *The Conquest of Lachish by Sennacherib,* Tel Aviv University, The Institute of Archaeology, 1982, p. 113, fig. 88.

p. 77: after
G. Zimmer, *Spiegel im Antikenmuseum,* Staatliche Museen Preussischer Kulturbesitz, Berlin 1987, p. 32, Abb. 18. Henceforth: Zimmer

p. 83: after
Zimmer, p. 31, Abb. 17.

p. 89: after
Erman, p. 198.

p. 90: after
Ch. Singer, E. Holmyard, A.R. Hall, *A History of Technology,* I, Clarendon Press, Oxford 1956, p. 291, fig. 188. Henceforth: Singer et al.

p. 93: after
Singer, et al., p. 292, fig. 189.

p. 94: after
Maiuri, p. 29.

p. 96 above: after
Singer, et al., p. 292, fig. 190.

p. 97 below: after
Daremberg, V, s.v. "Unguentum," p. 596, fig. 7234.

p. 113: after
Erman, p. 513.

p. 114: after
E. Naville, *Temple of Deir el Bahari,* III, London 1898, pl. LXXIV. Henceforth: Naville

p. 115: after
Naville, pl. LXXVIII.

p. 116: after
*Encyclopaedia Biblica,* IV, Bialik Institute, Jerusalem 1962, s.v. "Levonah," p. 418 (Hebrew).

p. 120: after
J. Feliks, *Plant World of the Bible,* Masada, Tel Aviv 1957, p. 253 (Hebrew).

p. 121: after
Naville, pl. LXXIX.

p. 125: after
Richter & Milne, p. 15.

## Abbreviations

*AJA*
*American Journal of Archaeology*

*BA*
*Biblical Archaeologist*

*IEJ*
*Israel Exploration Journal*

*JEA*
*Journal of Egyptian Archaeology*

*JGS*
*Journal of Glass Studies*

*JHS*
*Journal of Hellenic Studies*

*JJS*
*Journal of Jewish Studies*

*JNES*
*Journal of Near Eastern Studies*

*QDAP*
*Quarterly of the Department of Antiquities in Palestine*

*PEQ*
*Palestine Exploration Quarterly*

## Bibliography

*Egypt's Golden Age: The Art of Living in the New Kingdom 1558-1085 B.C.,* Museum of Fine Arts, Boston 1982, pp. 184–227.

A. Erman, *Life in Ancient Egypt,* New York 1971, pp. 218–233.

R.J. Forbes, *Studies in Ancient Technology,* III, Leiden 1965², pp. 6–20; 30–43.

S. Krauss, *Talmudische Archäologie,* I, Hildesheim 1966, pp. 190–198, 209–244.

A. Lucas, revised by J.R. Harris, *Ancient Egyptian Materials and Industries,* London 1962⁴, pp. 80–90.

J. Preuss, *Biblisch-Talmudische Medizin,* Berlin 1911, pp. 429–434, 617–642.

Ch. Singer, E.J. Holmyard, A.R. Hall, *A History of Technology,* I, Oxford 1956, pp. 260–261; 285–292.

Uza Zevulun, Yael Olenik, *Function and Design in the Talmudic Period,* Haaretz Museum, 2nd ed., Tel Aviv 1979.

## Body Care

Ruth Amiran, *Museum Haaretz Bulletin* 14· (1972), pp. 67–77.

Ruth Amiran, *JNES* 21 (1962), pp. 161–174.

I. Ben-Dor, *QDAP* 11 (1944), pp. 93–112.

V. Fritz, *BA* 50 (1987), pp. 232–240.

R. Ginouvés, *Balaneutiké, Recherches sur le bain dans l'antiquité grecque,* Paris 1962.

Ch. F. Jean, *Archiv Orientální* 17 (1949), pp. 320–329.

Th. Klausen, ed., *Reallexikon für Antike und Christentum,* I, 1950, s.v. Bad.

S. Laser, *Medizin und Körperpflege,* Göttingen 1983, pp. 138–172.

B. Meissner, *Babylonien und Assyrien,* I, Heidelberg 1920, pp. 411–413.

Marjorie J. Milne, *AJA* 48 (1944), pp. 26–38.

O.W. Muscarella, *Expedition* 16 (1974), pp. 25–29.

A. Neuberger, *The Technical Arts and Sciences of the Ancients,* London 1930, pp. 110–121.

E. Neufeld, *BA* 34 (1971), pp. 42–66.

R. Reich, *JJS* 39 (1988), pp. 102–107.

J. Vandier d'Abbadie, *Les objets de toilette égyptiens au Musée du Louvre,* Paris 1972.

H. Weippert, *Biblisches Reallexikon,* s.v. Bad und Baden, Tübingen 1977.

Bibliography

## Facial Care and Makeup

D. Barag, *JGS* 17 (1975), pp. 23–36.

D. Barag, *JGS* 24 (1982), pp. 11–19.

B. Brandl, *Anatolian Studies* 34 (1984), pp. 15–41.

Malka Hershkovitz, *IEJ* 36 (1986), pp. 45–51.

J.R. Partington, *Origins and Development of Applied Chemistry,* London 1935.

Holly Pittman, *Art of the Bronze Age, Southeastern Iran, Western Central Asia, and the Indus Valley,* The Metropolitan Museum of Art, New York 1984, pp. 43–47.

R.A. Stucky, *Dedalo* 19 (1974), pp. 94–99.

R. Campbell Thompson, *Dictionary of Assyrian Chemistry and Geology,* Oxford 1936, pp. 49–51.

J. Vandier d'Abbadie, *Les objets de toilette égyptiens au Musée du Louvre,* Paris 1972.

I. Wallert, *Der Verzierte Löffel, Seine Formgeschichte und Verwendung im Alten Ägypten,* Wiesbaden 1967.

Virginia Webb, *Levant* 4 (1972), pp. 148–155.

H.E. Winlock, *The Treasures of Three Egyptian Princesses,* The Metropolitan Museum of Art, New York 1948.

## Hair and Hair-styles

D. Balsdon, *Antike Welt* 10 (3) (1979), pp. 40–56.

J. Carcopino, *Daily Life in Ancient Rome,* London 1946, pp. 157–169.

J. S. Cox, *JEA* 63 (1977), pp. 67–70.

K. Galling, *Biblisches Reallexikon,* Tübingen 1977, s.v. Haartracht.

A. Koester, *Burlington Magazine* 13 (1908), pp. 351–358.

B. Meissner, *Babylonien und Assyrien,* I, Heidelberg 1920, pp. 410–411.

Elizabeth Riefstahl, *JNES* 15 (1956), pp. 10–17.

## Mirrors

J.D. Cooney, *Bulletin of the Cleveland Museum of Art* 60 (1973), pp. 215–221.

Ch. Lilyquist, *Ancient Egyptian Mirrors from the Earliest Times through the Middle Kingdom,* München 1979.

W.M.F. Petrie, *Objects of Daily Use,* Guildford 1974, pp. 28–33.

Nancy Thomson de Grummond, ed., *A Guide to Etruscan Mirrors,* Tallahassee 1982.

Gisela Zahlhaas, *Römische Reliefspiegel,* München 1975.

G. Zimmer, *Spiegel im Antikenmuseum,* Berlin 1987.

## Perfume Production

N. Avigad, *Discovering Jerusalem,* Jerusalem 1980, pp. 129–131.

D. Barag, *IEJ* 22 (1972), pp. 24–26.

A. Basch, *IEJ* 22 (1972), pp. 27–32.

E. Ebeling, *Orientalia* 17 (1948), pp. 143–144, 299–313; 19 (1950), pp. 17–19.

P. Faure, *Parfums et Aromates de l'Antiquité,* Mesnil-sur-l'Estrée 1987.

B. Mazar, Trude Dothan, I. Dunayevsky, *Atiqot* 5 (1966), pp. 1–100.

E. Paszthory, *Antike Welt* 2 (1988), pp. 3–20.

J. Patrich & B. Arubas, *IEJ* 39 (1989), pp. 43–59.

C.W. Shelmerdine, *The Perfume Industry of Mycenaean Pylos,* Göteborg 1985.

M. Zohary, *Plants of the Bible,* Cambridge 1982.

## The Spice Trade

M. Broshi, *JJS* 38 (1987), pp. 31–37.

D.M. Dixon, *JEA* 55 (1969), pp. 55–65.

M. Elat, *Economic Relations in the Lands of the Bible c. 1000–539 B.C.,* Jerusalem 1977.

N. Glueck, *BASOR* 71 (1938), pp. 16–17.

N. Groom, *Frankincense and Myrrh, A Study of the Arabian Incense Trade,* London 1981.

J. I. Miller, *The Spice Trade of the Roman Empire 29BC to AD 641,* Oxford 1969.

W. W. Müller, *Proceedings of the Seminar for Arabian Studies* 6 (1976), pp. 124–136.

H. Ogino, *Orient* 3 (1967), pp. 21–39.

Y. Shiloh, *PEQ* 119 (1987), pp. 9–18.

S.E. Sidebotham, *Roman Economic Policy in the Erythra Thalassa 30 B.C–217 A.D,* Leiden 1986.

A. Tscherikower, *Mizraim* 4–5 (1937), pp. 25–90.

Gus W. Van Beek & A. Jamme, *BASOR* 151 (1958), pp. 9–15.

Gus W. Van Beek, *BA* 23 (1960), pp. 70–95.

Gus W. Van Beek, *Scientific American,* December 1969, pp. 36–46.

Gus W. Van Beek, *Archaeology* 36 (1983), p. 19.

Y. Yadin, *BASOR* 196 (1969), pp. 37–45.

## Spices in Funerary Customs

Virginia R. Anderson-Stojanovic, *AJA* 91 (1987), pp. 105–122.

D. Barag, *IEJ* 22 (1972), pp. 24–26.

G. Barkay, *Ketef Hinnom – A Treasure Facing Jerusalem's Walls,* The Israel Museum, Jerusalem 1986.

R. Hachlili, *PEQ* 115 (1983), pp. 115–132.

S. Klein, *Tod und Begräbnis in Palästina zur Zeit der Tannaiten,* Berlin 1908.

Donna C. Kurtz & J. Boardman, *Greek Burial Customs,* London 1971.

E. Meyers, *Jewish Ossuaries, Reburial and Rebirth,* Rome 1971.

L.Y. Rahmani, *BA* 44 (1981), pp. 171–177; 220–235; 45 (1982), pp. 43–53; 109–119.

E. Stern, in *The World History of the Jewish People, The Age of the Monarchies: Culture and Society,* ed. A. Malamat, Jerusalem 1979, pp. 270–278.

E. Stern, *Material Culture of the Land of the Bible in the Persian Period 538–332 B.C.,* Jerusalem 1982, pp. 125–127.

J.M.C. Toynbee, *Death and Burial in the Roman World,* London 1982.

D. Zlotnick, *The Tractate "Mourning" (Semahot),* New Haven and London 1966.